!7

Fatigue in Multiple Sclerosis
A Guide to Diagnosis and Management

Fatigue in Multiple Sclerosis
A Guide to Diagnosis and Management

Lauren B. Krupp, M.D.

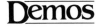

New York

Demos Medical Publishing Inc., 368 Park Avenue South, New York, New York
10016

Made in the United States of America

Library of Congress Cataloging-in-Publication Data

Krupp, Lauren B.
  Fatigue in multiple sclerosis : a guide to diagnosis and management /
Lauren B. Krupp.
      p. ; cm.
  Includes bibliographical references and index.
  ISBN 1-888799-81-1 (pbk. : alk. paper)
  1. Fatigue.   2. Multiple sclerosis—Complications.
  [DNLM: 1. Multiple Sclerosis—complications.   2. Fatigue—etiology.
3. Fatigue—therapy.   WL 360 K94f 2004]   I. Title.
  RB150.F37.K783 2004
  616.8'34—dc22
                                                          2004001625

The book is dedicated to individuals with MS and the family, friends, and professionals who participate in their care.

CONTENTS

PREFACE

It has been over 20 years since the first reports on fatigue began to demonstrate the extraordinary prevalence and impact of this symptom on multiple sclerosis (MS) patients. In the past two decades, our knowledge of MS-related fatigue and its consequences has improved dramatically. Studies in the area of MS-related fatigue have revealed several theories about its pathophysiologic basis, including alterations in immune and endocrine system activity, neuronal damage, hypofunctionality of certain areas of the brain, and psychological factors such as mood disorders and poor coping skills. Ample research studies have been published that support the contribution of the various biologic and psychologic factors underlying fatigue. However, it is unlikely that any one of these factors, standing alone, is the sole cause of fatigue in any individual. It is far more likely that there is a complex set of interactions among these factors, with each contributing in some manner to the onset of fatigue and its severity.

The goals of this book are: 1) to discuss the definitions of fatigue and illustrate its high frequency in MS; 2) to familiarize the MS care provider with the tools available to diagnose MS fatigue; and finally 3) to bring together the knowledge that has been generated about the treatment of fatigue. Along with the recognition of the impact of MS-related fatigue, there has been progress in different pharmacologic and nonpharmacologic approaches to treatment. The book also reveals several areas in which continued research is needed.

It is my hope that the reader of this book takes away the message that fatigue is a condition for which interventions are possible. Neither the patient nor the physician should feel resigned to its inevitability. Various therapies, support systems, and treatment of underlying affective disorders can be beneficial for fatigue and thereby favorably influence quality of life.

ACKNOWLEDGMENTS

Thank you Alexa, Gina, and Kara for all your help. I am grateful to Harold Schombert for his incredible assistance and appreciate the patience and support of Dr. Diana M. Schneider. I am also grateful to Monique, and to Teva Neuroscience for its interest in this topic and its support in the form of an educational grant.

Fatigue in Multiple Sclerosis

A Guide to Diagnosis and Management

CHAPTER 1
Introduction

The word "fatigue" does not lend itself easily to interpretation. Ask healthcare providers form various specialties to define fatigue, and you will likely come up with a wide range of terms, including muscle tiredness, exhaustion, sleepiness, weakness, depression, languor, and any number of others. The phenomenon of "fatigue" cannot be described with complete accuracy in all cases, and appreciation of fatigue's importance or role in illness can vary with one's background.

Compounding the study and understanding of fatigue is that physicians usually rely solely on the patient's report of symptoms to make a diagnosis. Fatigue is almost always a subjective experience. Therefore, physicians may have various definitions in their own minds, any or none of which may mesh with the patient's own definition. Patients' self-perceptions of fatigue may be complicated to a great extent by confounding factors that are common among multiple sclerosis (MS) patients, including pain, depression, loss of cognitive skills, and "learned helplessness."

The identification of fatigue as a distinct clinical entity requires both art and science, and most of all a willingness and ability to listen carefully to patients and their families. Obtaining a comprehensive history requires a full understanding of the circumstances in which fatigue occurs (physical, cognitive, and psychosocial), and demands consideration of a large number of disorders, including anxiety, depression, excessive daytime sleepiness, pain, and spasticity, all of which may mimic or contribute to fatigue.

This is a challenge to the most experienced practitioner, but it is a challenge that must be undertaken with the MS patient because of the extraordinarily high frequency and severity of fatigue in MS. While recognized for many decades as a core feature of MS, many reports from the

1980s[1] and since have noted that fatigue occurs in 78% or more of MS patients and that it limits activity more than any other MS symptom. Fatigue has emerged as perhaps the single most frequent and often most disabling symptom of the disease.[1–5]

Fatigue can have a major impact on functioning and activities of daily living, quality of life, employment, and psychological well-being. The effects are not limited to the patient: The individual's family can suffer as well. Thus, each time the patient presents with new-onset fatigue or an increase in pre-existing fatigue, the physician must delve deeply into the patient's medication use (prescription, over-the-counter, and illicit), diet, exercise programs, activities of daily living, disease history, family history, psychiatric history, psychosocial support network, and the possibility of other disorders that may be causing fatigue to tease out the potential reasons for this symptom.

Unfortunately, all too often, the approach to the fatigue workup does not nearly approach this level of comprehensiveness. In fact, quite the opposite is usually true. Fatigue is often given little attention by physicians. This has been amply demonstrated not only in MS, but in other diseases. In one study of over 1,300 cancer patients, although 58% reported being "somewhat fatigued" or "very much fatigued," only 52% of those with fatigue ever reported it to their hospital physician, and only 14% had received treatment or advice about managing this symptom.[6]

While immune modulation, inflammation, demyelination, axonal transection, and brain hypometabolism all appear to play important roles in fatigue, other physical factors are strongly related to fatigue symptoms, including pain and deconditioning, as well as psychologic factors such as depression. Identifying fatigue clearly depends on what questions are asked, and what diagnostic criteria are used. It is often necessary to assess patients for the presence or absence of potential overlapping or confounding symptoms.

This book is intended to be a practical guide to physicians and other health care providers interested in better understanding MS-associated fatigue. The topics cover the impact of fatigue on the individual with MS, the potential etiologies underlying MS-related fatigue, workup and diagnosis, and pharmacologic and nonpharmacologic management strategies. More than many other symptom physicians treat, the problem of fatigue—and indeed, therapeutic efforts for the MS patient in general—is a team effort, requiring the expertise of the nursing staff, physical, occupational, and psychotherapists, social work providers, nutritionists, and the patient's family and friends. The goal of this book is to provide information that is valuable to the many different health care providers involved in the care of the individual with MS.

References

1. Freal JE, Kraft GH, Coryell JK. Symptomatic fatigue in multiple sclerosis. *Arch Phys Med Rehabil.* 1984;65:135-138.
2. Bakshi R, Shaikh ZA, Miletich RS, et al. Fatigue in multiple sclerosis and its relationship to depression and neurologic disability. *Mult Scler.* 2000;6:181-185.
3. Krupp LB, Alvarez LA, LaRocca NG, Scheinberg LC. Fatigue in multiple sclerosis. *Arch Neurol.* 1988;45:435-437.
4. Bergamaschi R, Romani A, Versino M, Poli R, Cosi V. Clinical aspects of fatigue in multiple sclerosis. *Funct Neurol.* 1997;12:247-251.
5. Fisk JD, Pontefract A, Ritvo PG, Archibald CJ, Murray TJ. The impact of fatigue on patients with multiple sclerosis. *Can J Neurol Sci.* 1994;21:9-14.
6. Stone P, Richards M, A'Hern R, Hardy J. A study to investigate the prevalence, severity and correlates of fatigue among patients with cancer in comparison with a control group of volunteers without cancer. *Ann Oncol.* 2000;11:561-567.

CHAPTER 2

What Is Multiple Sclerosis-Related Fatigue?

A 51-year-old man with relapsing-remitting multiple sclerosis (MS) presented to the MS center with symptoms of severe fatigue, leg pain, and hip pain. He has been on immunomodulator therapy for 5 years. His symptoms had been continuing without remission for 1 month. He was employed as an executive in a construction firm. Although he was still working, he was beginning to consider going on disability.

His neurologic examination showed increased tone in his right leg and additional weakness of the iliopsoas (hip flexors) and hamstring muscles on that side. A magnetic resonance imaging (MRI) scan showed no new lesions in the spinal cord or brain, and urinalysis and urine culture were negative for infection or bacterial growth. The patient's pain improved with the addition of physical therapy and an antispasticity agent taken at bedtime. He reported a major improvement in pain and some improvement in fatigue, but was still dissatisfied with how tired he felt in the early afternoon.

The neurologist was pleased with the overall improvement in the patient's response to physical therapy and failed to make recommendations for managing the fatigue. The patient in turn reported his concerns to the nurse. He explained how fatigue was negatively impacting his career, and how his employer was critical of the patient's slowness in getting things done. He also expressed his concern that both his physician and his boss thought his fatigue was "laziness," and that "no one understood his MS."

As the above case shows, fatigue can be a difficult concept to communicate from both the provider's and the patient's standpoint.

Because "fatigue" is a common lay term, there can be a wide variation in the way that patients understand it, as well as in the way they understand related terms such as depression, weakness, deconditioning, tiredness, pain, and motivation. As diagnosing fatigue relies heavily on patient self-reporting, providers' recognition of fatigue can be limited by patients' inability to describe their symptoms accurately. At the same time, providers' own poor understanding of fatigue can contribute to a failure to diagnose fatigue. Providers are generally not trained to diagnose or even look for fatigue, and they usually underestimate its importance.

Because the word "fatigue" is laden with ambiguity, when patients come to physicians with complaints of fatigue, it is essential for physicians to determine accurately what patients mean by this complaint. It is equally important for providers to recognize when fatigue is present in cases where patients do not specifically complain of the symptom. Fatigue as a symptom incorporates a number of different concepts that have been applied and studied in a range of contexts.[1-5] Some of the more common associations with the word fatigue include:

- Physical tiredness;
- Mental tiredness;
- Lack of motivation;
- Difficulty concentrating;
- Inability to complete tasks;
- Feelings of depression;
- Feelings of anxiety;
- Failure to feel refreshed after sleep;
- Overall muscle weakness;
- Weakness in certain muscle groups;
- Poor performance at home or work;
- Performance that fails to meet prior expectations;
- Pain or physical discomfort; and
- Sleep difficulties.

One of the most challenging issues in defining fatigue is that there are few, if any, objective criteria that can aid physicians in observing fatigue for themselves. Other than certain cases of muscle weakness, which can be quantified through neuromuscular testing,[6] the definition of fatigue relies heavily on the patient's experience and the information that he or she can provide. Therefore, providers must always be respectful of patients' descriptions of their fatigue.

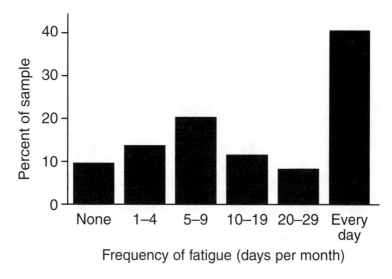

FIGURE 1   Frequency of fatigue problems during the past 30 days for MS patients. Source: Fisk JD et al. *Can J Neurol Sci.* 1994;21:9-14.[7]

Insufficient work has been performed in the area of defining fatigue. This is a little disappointing and is also surprising, given both the pervasiveness of fatigue in the MS population and its effects on daily functioning. Multiple sclerosis-related fatigue has been shown to be both highly prevalent and long lasting. More than 40% of 85 MS patients in one study reported feeling fatigued on every day of the month (Figure 1).[7]

Defining MS-Related Fatigue

A variety of investigations have ascribed different definitions to MS-related fatigue, including a feeling of tiredness that is out of proportion to the level of exertion, a feeling of weakness, the lack of capacity to generate sufficient muscle force,[1,2] or the lack of ability to sustain mental performance.[8] In 1998, the Multiple Sclerosis Council for Clinical Practice Guidelines published a consensus definition of fatigue. The Council, which was composed of a wide variety of MS providers, including neurologists, psychologists, rehabilitation therapists, and MS nurses, defined fatigue as:

> *A subjective lack of physical and/or mental energy that is perceived by the individual or caregiver to interfere with usual and desired activities.*[9]

The Council cited a number of advantages in this definition of fatigue, including the fact that it is a generalized definition that is easily understandable by MS patients as well as providers. Observing that the severity of fatigue may wax or wane depending on circumstances (e.g., physical exertion, the presence of infection, or hot weather), the Council separated chronic fatigue from acute fatigue. Under the Council's definition, chronic persistent fatigue was defined as:

- *Fatigue that is present for any amount of time on 50% of the days for more than 6 weeks.*
- *Fatigue that limits functional activities or quality of life.*

Acute fatigue was defined as:

- *New or a significant increase in feelings of fatigue in the previous 6 weeks.*
- *Fatigue that limits functional activities or quality of life.*

In addition to distinguishing between acute and chronic fatigue, providers should distinguish between fatigue that results from other MS symptoms (e.g., poor sleep, pain) and fatigue that is primarily due to the MS itself. Not infrequently, fatigue has multiple causes in the same individual. Strong lines of evidence suggest that fatigue is a primary disorder, directly related to the underlying pathophysiologic processes of MS itself, including immune dysregulation, inflammation, neuronal dysfunction, and demyelination. Factors that support the concept of fatigue as an inherent component of MS include: 1) the marked association between MS fatigue and heat; 2) the fact that fatigue may precede disease relapses or be a prominent symptom within a relapse; and 3) the observation that fatigue may be the first presenting symptom of MS.[10] When fatigue occurs secondary to other MS-related factors, frequent culprits are deconditioning, pain, poor sleep, and agents used to treat other symptoms of MS (e.g., muscle relaxants, anticonvulsants, and interferon betas).

It is also important for the provider to distinguish between "normal" and "abnormal" fatigue. Everyone feels fatigued at some point, and the problem is not necessarily related to MS. As many as 23% of the general population have experienced persistent fatigue at some point.[11] It is likely that fatigue appears along a continuum, in much the same way that blood pressure does, with some patients experiencing low levels of fatigue, some extremely high levels, and the remainder feeling "normal" levels (Figure 2).[12] The challenge to providers, therefore, is to determine not only when fatigue is present, but when it is pathologic. It has been suggested

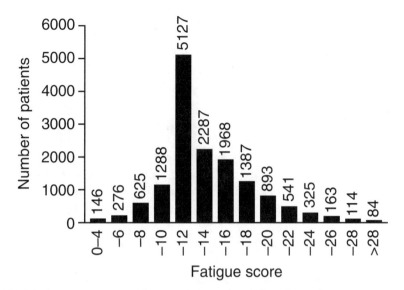

FIGURE 2 Dimensions of fatigue in a population-based sample.
Source: Pawlikowska T et al. *Br Med J.* 1994;308:763-766.[12]

that fatigue in normal individuals can be distinguished from MS-related fatigue based on the fact that MS-related fatigue:

• Worsens with heat;
• Prevents sustained physical activity;
• Interferes with physical functioning;
• Interferes with role performance;
• Emerges easily;
• Causes frequent problems; and
• Interferes with meeting one's responsibilities.[10]

Epidemiology and Impact of Fatigue in the MS Population

A variety of surveys and clinical studies have shown that fatigue is a major symptom, and highly prevalent in a number of disorders, including chronic fatigue syndrome, systemic lupus erythematosus, epilepsy, Parkinson's disease, and cancer. Much of what we have learned about fatigue over the past 2 decades, however, is attributable to work in the field of MS.[13] Fatigue in MS was not readily recognized or discussed before the early 1980s. In 1984, a seminal study on MS symptoms in 656 MS patients showed that fatigue was the single most commonly reported symptom, cited by 78% of patients.[14] The prevalence of fatigue was higher than "typical" MS symptoms such as difficulty in balance, tremor, gait disturbances, weakness, tingling/numbness, and bowel/bladder difficulties (Table 1).[14] The finding at this time was relatively novel; as based on the prior literature, the researchers did not expect fatigue to be a frequent symptom. Twenty-two percent of the patients reported that fatigue caused them to reduce their level of physical activity, 14% said it required them to have more rest, and 10% said that it forced them to quit work.[14]

Since that time, a number of studies have confirmed and expanded on the epidemiology of fatigue in the MS population and its potential associations with demographic characteristics, disease subtype, level of disability, emotional status, and other symptoms of MS. Fatigue has consistently been ranked among the most prevalent and disabling MS symptoms. In a 1997 United Kingdom MS Society survey of 233 persons with MS, 86% of patients reported symptoms of fatigue, more than balance problems (73%), muscle weakness (69%), and bladder/bowel problems

TABLE 1 Symptoms Reported by a Sample of 656 MS Patients

Symptom	No ADL Difficulty (%)	Producing ADL Difficulty (%)
Fatigue	22	56
Balance problems	24	50
Weakness/paralysis	18	45
Numbness/tingling/other sensory disturbance	39	24
Bladder problems	25	34
Increased muscle tension (spasticity)	23	26
Bowel problems	19	20
Difficulty remembering	21	16
Depression	18	18
Pain	15	21
Laugh or cry easily (emotional lability)	24	8
Double or blurred vision, partial or complete blindness	14	16
Shaking tremor	14	13
Speech and/or communication difficulties	12	11
Difficulty solving problems	12	9

ADL = activities of daily living.
Source: Freal JE et al. *Arch Phys Med Rehabil.* 1984;65:135-138.[14]

(66%).[15] Two thirds of MS patients have rated fatigue as one of the three worst symptoms of their disease.[10] It commonly occurs as the principal presenting symptom of the disease.[10]

Multiple sclerosis-related fatigue has also been contrasted with the fatigue experienced by either healthy adults or individuals with other medical disorders. The fatigue associated with MS is unique from that of healthy individuals in its disabling effect on activities of daily living, including carrying out physical activities and meeting one's responsibilities, as well as in its severity and frequency.[10,16] Qualitatively, MS-related fatigue is different from the fatigue associated with other medical conditions because of its aggravation by heat.

Part of the difficulty in recognizing fatigue in the MS patient is the fact that it does not correlate well with demographic characteristics, the clinical form of MS, or other MS signs and symptoms. For example, fatigue has not been found to correlate closely with either age or Expanded Disability Status Scale (EDSS) score,[17,18] and does not correlate with the level of disease activity as found on MRI.[19,20] In addition, there does not appear to be an association between fatigue and gender in MS patients.[21,22] The lack of association with these factors makes fatigue difficult to predict.

Nevertheless, fatigue *has* been found to be associated with perceived general and mental health,[7,23] and to have a substantial impact on activities. For example, fatigue has been shown to be a frequent cause of unemployment in MS patients.[24] It also limits social relationships and the ability to engage in self-care activities,[21] and generally limits the patient's ability to perform tasks requiring physical effort.[7] Fatigue may worsen some of the other symptoms of MS.[25] Some data have suggested that fatigue may be associated with older age and progressive forms of MS, as opposed to relapsing forms.[21,22] In one epidemiologic study of 368 individuals with MS from Norway, fatigue showed a significant inverse correlation with years of education and, for patients with progressive MS, positively correlated with age and disease duration.[26] Sleep disorders also are associated with fatigue.[3] Fatigue has been shown to be associated with overall decrements in quality of life on instruments that include assessments of health, job activity, housing, finances, and family and friendships.[27] The patient's sense of control over his or her symptoms also has been shown to be significantly associated with fatigue (Figure 3).[28]

One of the most consistent associations that has been observed is the association between fatigue and affective disorders, including depression and anxiety.[29] Studies have shown that anxiety and depression both

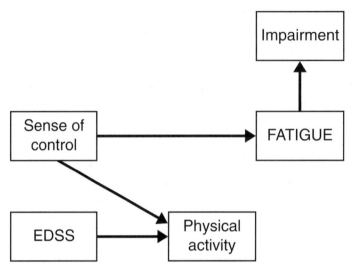

FIGURE 3   Fatigue model for MS, indicating effect of sense of control on fatigue and physical activity. Source: Vercoulen JHMM et al. *J Psychosom Res.* 1998;45:507-517.[28]

have a high positive predictive value and specificity for fatigue (approximately 80%),[3] and both depression and fatigue have been shown to have an impact on physical and mental health.[29] Despite this overlap, however, psychiatric involvement is present in a relatively small population of fatigued patients, and depression in itself, without fatigue, can be an independent predictor of poor quality of life.[30] For example, in a study of MS patients with severe fatigue, defined by a score on the Fatigue Severity Scale (FSS) of ≥4.0, very few patients had any evidence of major depression, as assessed by a psychiatric interview.[31] Thus, it is important to be aware that fatigue is generally an independent entity in the MS patient, and is rarely associated exclusively with psychiatric problems.[3] In those MS patients who are depressed, treatment of the depression should precede therapy for fatigue, to see if the fatigue resolves with the alleviation of mood symptoms.

Conclusions

The symptom of fatigue in the MS patient is one that incorporates a number of concepts, including weakness, tiredness, lack of motivation, affective disorders, pain, and sleepiness. Providers must be aware of all of these facets of fatigue, and any of these complaints should raise the index of suspicion for MS-related fatigue. Publication of a consensus definition of MS-related fatigue[9] has increased focus on this symptom. Because of the high prevalence of fatigue in MS patients, the presence of fatigue should be suspected unless and until it is specifically ruled out. Fatigue in MS is poorly related to disease type, disability level, gender, age, and imaging findings on MRI. Therefore, the provider must rely heavily on the patient's self-report in the diagnosis.

References

1. Schwid SR, Thornton CA, Pandya S, et al. Quantitative assessment of motor fatigue and strength in MS. *Neurology.* 1999;53:743-750.
2. Sheean GL, Murray NMF, Rothwell JC, Miller DH, Thompson AJ. An electrophysiological study of the mechanism of fatigue in multiple sclerosis. *Brain.* 1997;120:299-315.
3. Iriarte J, Subira ML, de Castro P. Modalities of fatigue in multiple sclerosis: correlation with clinical and biological factors. *Mult Scler.* 2000;6:124-130.
4. Holley S. Cancer-related fatigue: suffering a different fatigue. *Cancer Practice.* 2000;8:87-95.
5. Knowles G. Survey of nurses' assessment of cancer-related fatigue. *Eur J Cancer Care.* 2000;9:105-113.
6. Kent-Braun JA, LeBlanc R. Quantitation of central activation failure during maximal voluntary contractions in humans. *Muscle Nerve.* 1996;19:861-869.
7. Fisk JD, Pontefract A, Ritvo PG, Archibald CJ, Murray TJ. The impact of fatigue on patients with multiple sclerosis. *Can J Neurol Sci.* 1994;21:9-14.
8. Krupp LB, Elkins LE. Fatigue and declines in cognitive functioning in multiple sclerosis. *Neurology.* 2000;55:934-939..
9. MS Council for Clinical Practice Guidelines. *Fatigue in Multiple Sclerosis.* Washington, DC: Paralyzed Veterans Association; 1998.
10. Krupp LB, Alvarez LA, LaRocca NG, Scheinberg LC. Fatigue in multiple sclerosis. *Arch Neurol.* 1988;45:435-437.
11. Price RK, North CS, Wessely S, Fraser VJ. Estimating the prevalence of chronic fatigue syndrome and associated symptoms in the community. *Pub Health Reports.* 1992;107:514-522.
12. Pawlikowska T, Chandler T, Hirsch SR, et al. Population-based study of fatigue and distress. *Br Med J.* 1994;308:763-766.
13. Krupp LB. *Fatigue: The Most Common Complaints.* Philadelphia, PA: Elsevier Science; 2003.
14. Freal JE, Kraft GH, Coryell JK. Symptomatic fatigue in multiple sclerosis. *Arch Phys Med Rehabil.* 1984;65:135-138.
15. UK Multiple Sclerosis Society. *Symptom Management Survey Multiple Sclerosis.* 1997.
16. Krupp LB, LaRocca NG, Muir-Nash J, Steinberg AD. The Fatigue Severity Scale: application to patients with multiple sclerosis and systemic lupus erythematosus. *Arch Neurol.* 1989;46:1121-1123.
17. Kurtzke JF. Rating neurologic impairment in multiple sclerosis: an expanded disability status scale (EDSS). *Neurology.* 1983;33:1444-1452.
18. Murray TJ. Amantadine therapy for fatigue in multiple sclerosis. *Can J Neurol Sci.* 1985;12:251-254.

19. Bakshi R, Miletich RS, Hanschel K, et al. Fatigue in multiple sclerosis: cross-sectional correlation with brain MRI findings in 71 patients. *Neurology.* 1999;53:1151-1153.

20. Mainero C, Faroni J, Gasperini C, et al. Fatigue and magnetic resonance imaging activity in multiple sclerosis. *J Neurol.* 1999;246:454-458.

21. Iriarte J, Katsamakis G, de Castro P. The Fatigue Descriptive Scale (FDS): a useful tool to evaluate fatigue in multiple sclerosis: *Mult Scler.* 1999;5:10-16.

22. Colosimo C, Millefiorini E, Grasso MG, et al. Fatigue in MS is associated with specific clinical features. *Acta Neurol Scand.* 1995;92:353-355.

23. Monks J. Experiencing symptoms in chronic illness: fatigue in multiple sclerosis. *Int Disabil Studies.* 1989;11:78-83.

24. Scheinberg L, Holland N, La Rocca N, Laitin P, Bennett A, Hall H. Multiple sclerosis: earning a living. *N Y State J Med.* 1980;80:1395-1400.

25. Tola MA, Yugueros MI, Fernandez-Buey N, Fernandez-Herranz R. Impact of fatigue in multiple sclerosis: study of a population-based series in Valladolid (Spanish). *Revista de Neurologia.* 1998;26:930-933.

26. Lerdal A, Celius EG, Moum T. Fatigue and its association with sociodemographic variables among multiple sclerosis patients. *Mult Scler.* 2003;9:509-514.

27. Aronson K. Quality of life among persons with multiple sclerosis and their caregivers. *Neurology.* 1997;48:74-80.

28. Vercoulen JHMM, Swanink CMA, Galama JMD, et al. The persistence of fatigue in chronic fatigue syndrome and multiple sclerosis: development of a model. *J Psychosom Res.* 1998;45:507-517.

29. Bakshi R, Shaikh ZA, Miletich RS, et al. Fatigue in multiple sclerosis and its relationship to depression and neurologic disability. *Mult Scler.* 2000;6:181-185.

30. Amato MP, Ponziani G, Rossi F, Liedl CL, Stefanile C, Rossi L. Quality of life in multiple sclerosis: the impact of depression, fatigue and disability. *Mult Scler.* 2001;7:340-344.

31. Pepper CM, Krupp LB, Friedberg F, Doscher C, Coyle PK. A comparison of neuropsychiatric characteristics in chronic fatigue syndrome, multiple sclerosis, and major depression. *J Neuropsychiatry Clin Neurosci.* 1993;5:200-205.

CHAPTER 3
The Measurement of Fatigue

A great deal of attention has been focused on the accurate identification and measurement of fatigue in the past 20 years.[1] Different scales and techniques have been developed not only to attempt to differentiate the pathologic fatigue of multiple sclerosis (MS) from fatigue of healthy individuals and that experienced by patients with other disorders, but also to distinguish fatigue from related MS symptoms such as excessive daytime sleepiness or depression.

While measurement techniques vary considerably, they all fall into one of two categories. *Subjective fatigue measurement scales* endeavor to measure patients' perceived level of fatigue by asking them to self-report the existence of fatigue and/or fatigue severity. The consensus definition of MS fatigue proffered by the MS Council for Clinical Practice Guidelines is an example of the subjective fatigue that these scales endeavor to capture. The consensus definition states that MS fatigue is a "subjective lack of physical and or mental energy that is perceived by the individual or caregiver to interfere with usual or desired activities."[2] *Objective fatigue measurement scales* endeavor to quantify the patient's level of fatigue through various parameters such as a reduction in muscle force generation over a specific period of exertion, or an increase in error rate or time necessary to complete a cognitive/neuropsychological testing task that requires sustained vigilance. Each approach to fatigue measurement has advantages and drawbacks.

Subjective Measures of Fatigue

Fatigue questionnaires in the form of self-report scales are the most widely used methods of measuring fatigue, and have been the tools employed in most clinical investigations. These scales, all of which measure the patient's perceived level of fatigue, have a number of advantages that make them useful for clinical practice. They are generally short, are widely available, are easily understandable by the patient, and require little prior training by the health care provider and staff. The results can be expressed as a summary score or the mean of the individual question scores.

Self-report fatigue measures address core feelings of fatigue such as a sense of exhaustion or tiredness, as well as decreased motivation associated with the fatigue state and its accompanying negative affect. Additional components often included in measures of subjective fatigue are the duration and frequency of fatigue and the deleterious effect of fatigue on activities of daily living. While the content of different items varies among different scales, there is also a significant degree of item similarity across scales. The questionnaires range in length from unidimensional scales[3–6] to longer multidimensional assessments.[7–10]

With respect to scaling methods, the most common approach is to use a Likert format in which subjects are asked to report the degree to which they endorse a particular item (e.g., "feeling exhausted") on an ordered scale (e.g., ranging from 0=not at all to 5=completely) as a way of gauging the symptom's severity or intensity (see FSS, Table 1). Alternatively, subjects can be asked to bisect the line of a visual analogue scale (VAS) for the same purpose. The advantages of the Likert scale include its ease of scoring and better accessibility for respondents.[11,12]

Listed in Table 2 are a number of fatigue self-report scales of varying complexity, including the Visual Analog Scale for Fatigue (VAS-F);[4] the Fatigue Severity Scale (FSS);[3] the Fatigue Impact Scale (FIS);[10] the Modified Fatigue Impact Scale (MFIS),[2] which along with the FSS is widely used in studies of MS; the Fatigue Descriptive Scale (FDS);[13] and the Fatigue Scale (FS).[14] Additional measures such as the MS-Specific Fatigue Scale (MS-FS),[15] the Checklist of Individual Strength (CIS),[16] the Fatigue Assessment Instrument (FAI),[8] and the Fatigue Symptom Inventory (FSI)[17] have also been used, as have multiple other measures, including the Fatigue Symptom Checklist (FSC),[18,19] the Multidimensional Assessment of Fatigue (MAF),[20] the Multidimensional Fatigue Inventory (MFI),[7] the Multicomponent Fatigue Scale (MFS),[21] the Multidimensional Fatigue Symptom Inventory (MFSI),[9] the Piper Fatigue Scale (PFS),[11,22] and the Rochester Fatigue Diary (RFD).[23]

TABLE 1 The Fatigue Severity Scale

For each question, the patient is asked to choose a number from 1 to 7 that indicates how much she or he agrees with each statement, where 1 indicates strongly disagree and 7 indicates strongly agree.

Statement	Score
1. My motivation is lower when I am fatigued.	_____
2. Exercise brings on my fatigue.	_____
3. I am easily fatigued.	_____
4. Fatigue interferes with my physical functioning.	_____
5. Fatigue causes frequent problems for me.	_____
6. My fatigue prevents sustained physical functioning.	_____
7. Fatigue interferes with my carrying out certain duties and responsibilities.	_____
8. Fatigue is among my three most disabling symptoms.	_____
9. Fatigue interferes with my work, family, or social life.	_____
Total Score:	_____

Scoring is done by taking the average of the nine scores. A score of 4 or higher generally indicates severe fatigue.

Copyright © Lauren B. Krupp, MD.

In many cases, scales have been designed to assess fatigue in specific disease populations. For example, the FDS[13] and the MS-FS[15] ask questions about the effects of fatigue on heat, factors that are of particular importance to the MS patient, whereas the FSI was developed primarily for cancer-related fatigue.[17] Choosing a particular fatigue measure requires an understanding of the purpose of the investigation and the specific characteristics of the patient population of interest.

Subjective fatigue scales fall into two categories: *unidimensional*, which attempt to measure fatigue as a single construct, and *multidimensional*, which attempt to measure fatigue as several constructs or differentiate among various forms of fatigue (e.g., physical, cognitive, and psychosocial). Unidimensional scales range from the simple VAS-F to more complex measures such as the FSS, the fatigue subscale of the Profile of Mood States (POMS),[24] and the vitality subscale of the Medical Outcomes Survey Short Form 36 (SF-36).[25]

The VAS-F is a 50- or 100-cm line that asks patients to rate their level of fatigue on a scale of 0 (no fatigue) to 100 (fatigue as bad as can be) by marking their fatigue level on the line (Figure 1). The VAS-F has been used

TABLE 2 Some Fatigue Scales That Have Been Employed in MS and Other Populations

Scale	Author, Year	Initial Population	Specified Fatigue Subscales	Item Length	Item Scoring	Fatigue Time Frame Measured
Fatigue Symptom Checklist (FSC)	Kogi, 1970 (Japanese)[18]; Haylock, 1979 (English)[19]	Healthy (Koji); cancer (Haylock)	Drowsiness and dullness, projection of physical disintegration, difficulty in concentration	30	Yes/no	Now
Piper Fatigue Scale (PFS)	Piper, 1989[22] (revised in Piper, 1998)[11]	Cancer	Behavioral/severity, affective meaning, sensory, cognitive mood	22 (plus 5 open-ended questions)	0–10	1 item asks for duration
Fatigue Severity Scale (FSS)	Krupp, 1989[3]	MS, SLE, healthy	None	9	1–7	Not stated
Single-Item Visual Analog Scale (VAS) of Fatigue	Krupp, 1989[3]	MS, SLE, healthy	None	1	VAS	Not stated
Visual Analog Scale for Fatigue (VAS-F)	Lee, 1991[4]	Sleep disordered, healthy	Energy, fatigue	18	VAS	Not stated
Fatigue Assessment Instrument (FAI)	Schwartz, 1993[8]	Lyme disease, CFS, SLE, MS, dysthymia, healthy	Fatigue severity, situation specificity, consequences of fatigue, response to rest/sleep	29	1–7	Past 2 weeks

(continued on next page)

TABLE 2 Some Fatigue Scales That Have Been Employed in MS and Other Populations (continued)

Scale	Author, Year	Initial Population	Specified Fatigue Subscales	Item Length	Item Scoring	Fatigue Time Frame Measured
Fatigue Scale (FS)	Chalder, 1993[14]	Primary care	Physical, mental	14	Yes/no	Not stated
Checklist of Individual Strength (CIS)	Vercoulen, 1994[16]	CFS	Subjective experience of fatigue, concentration, motivation, physical activity	24	7-point scale	Not stated
Fatigue Impact Scale (FIS)	Fisk, 1994[10] (modified version [MFIS] by Multiple Sclerosis Council for Clinical Practice Guidelines, 1998)[2]	MS	Physical, cognitive, psychosocial	FIS: 40; MFIS: 21 (a 5-item short form is also available)	0–4	Past 4 weeks
Multidimensional Assessment of Fatigue (MAF)	Belza, 1995[20]	Rheumatoid arthritis	Degree, severity, distress, impact on activities of daily living	15	1–10	1 item asks for duration
Multidimensional Fatigue Inventory (MFI)	Smets, 1995[7]	Students, physicians, cancer, CFS	General fatigue, physical fatigue, mental fatigue, reduced motivation, reduced activity	20	1–7	Not stated
Multicomponent Fatigue Scale (MFS)	Paul, 1998[21]*	MS, myasthenia gravis	Mental, physical	15	0–5	At present and compared to recent past

(continued on next page)

19

TABLE 2 Some Fatigue Scales That Have Been Employed in MS and Other Populations (continued)

Scale	Author, Year	Initial Population	Specified Fatigue Subscales	Item Length	Item Scoring	Fatigue Time Frame Measured
Multidimensional Fatigue Symptom Inventory (MFSI)	Stein, 1998[9]	Cancer	Global, somatic, affective, behavioral, cognitive	83 (short form: 30)	0–4	Last week
Fatigue Descriptive Scale (FDS)	Iriarte, 1999[13]	MS	Spontaneous mention of fatigue, antecedent conditions, frequency, impact on life	5	0–3	Not stated
Fatigue Symptom Inventory (FSI)	Hann, 2000[17]	Cancer	Intensity, duration, impact on quality of life	13	0–10	Past week
Rochester Fatigue Diary (RFD)	Schwid, 2002[23]	MS	Lassitude (reduced energy)	12 (1 item 12 times over 24 hours)	VAS	Past 2 hours

*A variation on the Chalder Fatigue Scale.
MS=multiple sclerosis; SLE=systemic lupus erythematosus; CFS=chronic fatigue syndrome.

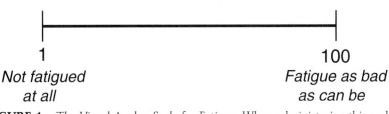

FIGURE 1 The Visual Analog Scale for Fatigue. When administering this scale, patients should be asked to mark their fatigue severity on the line, ranging from 0 (not fatigued at all) to 100 (fatigue as bad as can be).

in MS fatigue populations and has shown the ability to detect response to therapy.[26,27] It has the benefit of ease of use and interpretation, and easy translation into multiple languages. In addition, similar VAS scales can also be administered at the same time to ask patients to rate other symptoms such as pain. However, the VAS-F has drawbacks in that it may be less reliable than questionnaires and is more difficult for investigators to score. There is also the concern that a single response may be vulnerable to "impulsive answering," and answers may fluctuate, depending on situations such as time of day.

The FSS is a nine-item scale that assesses disabling fatigue in various medical populations (Table 1), and was developed as an improved method over the VAS-F. Like many of these scales, the FSS can be scored using the sum total of the responses, or be presented as the average score. The FSS has shown high reliability, validity, and internal consistency,[3] and has been the most widely used in cross-sectional and longitudinal studies of MS fatigue. It has also been shown to be effective for distinguishing fatigue in medically ill populations (systemic lupus erythematosus and MS) from those of healthy, nonfatigued controls, and like other scales, has shown the ability to detect positive effects of treatment.[3,15,27,28]

The scores of these various unidimensional fatigue scales may differ in subtle ways across different disorders. For example, it has been suggested that in the chronic fatigue syndrome (CFS) population, the FS focuses more on the intensity of fatigue, while the FSS assesses to a greater extent functional outcomes of fatigue.[29] In contrast, in studies of head trauma, the FIS may be more comprehensive than the FSS.[30]

A number of multidimensional scales have been developed in attempts to identify different forms of fatigue or analyze it across different domains (Table 2). Examples of scales designed to assess multiple dimensions, including social and physical functioning, include the FIS[10] and FDS,[13] as well as the MFI[7] and the MAF,[20] both of which have been used in a variety of disease groups, including arthritis, cancer, CFS, and pulmonary disease.

There are varying levels of support for the utility of these multidimensional measures. For example, the FDS was developed to discriminate between asthenia and fatigability, based on prior observations of the lack of correlation between muscle fatigue and perceived fatigue.[13] The FIS was designed to assess the perceived effect of fatigue on cognition, physical functioning, and psychosocial functioning (Table 3), based on the assumption that asking patients to measure the effect of fatigue on activ-

---

TABLE 3   The Fatigue Impact Scale

For each of the following statements, rate your score as a small problem (score of 1), moderate problem (2), big problem (3), or extreme problem (4).

Because of my fatigue:	**Score**	**Dimension**
1. I feel less alert.	_____	Cognitive
2. I feel that I am more isolated from social contact.	_____	Social
3. I have to reduce my workload or responsibilities.	_____	Social
4. I am more moody.	_____	Social
5. I have difficulty paying attention for a long period.	_____	Cognitive
6. I feel like I cannot think clearly.	_____	Cognitive
7. I work less effectively (both inside or outside of the home).	_____	Social
8. I have to rely more on others to help me or do things for me.	_____	Social
9. I have difficulty planning activities ahead of time.	_____	Social
10. I am more clumsy and uncoordinated.	_____	Physical
11. I find that I am more forgetful.	_____	Cognitive
12. I am more irritable and more easily angered.	_____	Social
13. I have to be careful about pacing my physical activities.	_____	Physical
14. I am less motivated to do anything that requires physical effort.	_____	Physical
15. I am less motivated to engage in social activities.	_____	Social
16. My ability to travel outside my home is limited.	_____	Social
17. I have trouble maintaining physical effort for long periods.	_____	Physical
18. I find it difficult to make decisions.	_____	Cognitive
19. I have few social contacts outside of my own home.	_____	Social
20. Normal day-to-day events are stressful to me.	_____	Social

(continued on next page)

TABLE 3 The Fatigue Impact Scale (continued)

For each of the following statements, rate your score as a small problem (score of 1), moderate problem (2), big problem (3), or extreme problem (4).

Because of my fatigue:	Score	Dimension
21. I am less motivated to do anything that requires thinking.	_____	Cognitive
22. I avoid situations that are stressful to me.	_____	Social
23. My muscles feel much weaker than they should.	_____	Physical
24. My physical discomfort is increased.	_____	Physical
25. I have difficulty dealing with anything new.	_____	Social
26. I am less able to finish tasks that require thinking.	_____	Cognitive
27. I feel unable to meet the demands that people place on me.	_____	Social
28. I am less able to provide financial support for myself and my family.	_____	Social
29. I engage in less sexual activity.	_____	Social
30. I find it difficult to organize my thoughts when I am doing things at home or at work.	_____	Cognitive
31. I am less able to complete tasks that require physical effort.	_____	Physical
32. I worry about how I look to other people.	_____	Physical
33. I am less able to deal with emotional issues.	_____	Social
34. I feel slowed down in my thinking.	_____	Cognitive
35. I find it hard to concentrate.	_____	Cognitive
36. I have difficulty participating fully in family activities.	_____	Social
37. I have to limit my physical activities.	_____	Physical
38. I require more frequent or longer periods of rest.	_____	Physical
39. I am not able to provide as much emotional support to my family as I should.	_____	Social
40. Minor difficulties seem like major difficulties.	_____	Social

The total points for each subgroup (physical, cognitive, social) and the entire questionnaire are summed. For the Cognitive subscale (10 questions) and Physical subscale (10 questions), the maximum scores are 40 for each. For the Social subscale (20 questions), the maximum score is 80.

Source: Fisk JD et al. *Clin Infect Dis*. 1994;18(suppl 1):S79-S83.[10]

ities is more sensitive than asking patients to simply rate their feelings of fatigue.[10,31] Validation studies have shown a high degree of internal consistency for evaluating fatigue in MS patients and those with CFS, as well as the ability to discriminate between fatigue in these two disease states, with CFS patients reporting a higher level of dysfunction related to fatigue symptoms on the FIS.[10] A modified version of this 40-item scale, with elimination of redundancies, is included in the Multiple Sclerosis Clinical Practice Guidelines for fatigue.[2]

Innovative Methods to Measure Subjective Fatigue

A number of innovative methods of fatigue self-reporting attempt to provide a more accurate assessment of fatigue. For example, ecological momentary assessment is a computerized, palmtop tool that assesses fatigue phenomena at various points throughout the day, and has been used to study fatigue in patients with CFS.[32] It has the advantage of using multiple repeated observations, which are typically made in the daily environments that patients inhabit. Patients are asked to respond to fatigue rating questionnaires using the palmtop device at several random moments throughout the day, as well as during certain events. Additional subjective instruments such as the Rochester Fatigue Diary ask patients to fill out a VAS for each hour of the day.[23]

Limitations of Subjective Fatigue Scales

Despite the advantages of assessing multiple aspects of fatigue, it has been suggested that multidimensional measures of fatigue may show less robust psychometric properties of reliability, validity, and responsiveness than unidimensional fatigue measures such as the fatigue subscale of the POMS.[33]

Both multidimensional and unidimensional scales have the same limitations in that they are subject to rater bias, as they ask the patient to make a retrospective assessment of fatigue over varying degrees of time. They also ask patients to rate their fatigue without clearly defining it; as a result, the physician can never be entirely clear whether the patient is commenting on the distinct symptom of fatigue,[23] as opposed to related factors such as depression, weakness, sleepiness, or pain. The scales all show varying degrees of fluctuation, with the VAS-F generally acknowledged as the most prone to variation.

In addition, even multidimensional scales do not provide a truly accurate assessment of social, cognitive, or physical functioning. Such factors can only be obtained by more extensive investigation into the patient's individual circumstances (e.g., by confirming work attendance through the patient's employer or assessing performance on neuropsychological tests). Such steps may be time-consuming and impractical and, in cases such as confirming work attendance, may infringe upon the patient's confidentiality rights.

Objective Measures of Fatigue

Objective, performance-based measures attempt to quantify the patient's level of fatigue. For the most part, such measures have been limited to the research arena, and clinical applications are not widespread. Measures have been used for both physical and mental (cognitive) fatigue.

Physical Fatigue

Several approaches have been used to measure physical fatigue objectively, with most focusing on declines in performance during sustained muscle activity. For example, a Fatigue Index (FI) has been developed that calculates the ratio between the integral of muscle strength decay over time and maximal voluntary contraction.[34] Testing this model in 30 patients with MS, four patients with CFS, and 13 healthy controls, researchers found a significantly higher FI in the MS patients compared with both the controls and the CFS patients. The FI correlated with the presence of pyramidal signs and worsened during relapses affecting the pyramidal tract, but not during relapses not involving the pyramidal tract.[34]

In studies of maximal force generation, patients with MS were shown to generate only about three quarters of the maximal force-generating capacity of their muscles compared with controls. During repeated exercise, the muscles of MS patients showed greater fatigability compared with controls, as measured by a greater decrease in force generation.[35] Multiple sclerosis subjects have also demonstrated significantly lower peak force and a faster decline in force than controls, as measured with motor-evoked potentials.[36]

Cognitive Fatigue

Objective testing has been used to identify a form of "cognitive fatigue" among MS patients, who have often reported that fatigue adversely affects their cognitive functioning.[37] Cognitive impairment can be disabling, with a detrimental impact on employment and social functioning.[38]

In general, routine measures of cognitive ability, as evaluated with a standard neuropsychological battery, show no significant correlation with fatigue.[39,40] Further evidence of the disassociation between routine measures of cognitive functioning and fatigue can be found in the lack of a treatment effect of medications used to reduce fatigue on neuropsychogical performance.[41]

However, different strategies have been used to examine the issue of cognitive fatigue or induced cognitive decline. A pilot study that tested cognitive performance following physical exertion failed to detect cognitive decline, and did not include a control group comparison.[42] Another study that did not use sustained cognitive tasks did not show a difference between MS patients and control participants,[21] while a third study that measured sustained attention did show decrements in performance over time in MS patients compared with controls, but the test did not include other aspects of cognitive functioning.[43]

A more promising approach to assess this potential relationship was demonstrated by measuring cognitive fatigue before and after the performance of a continuously effortful cognitive task.[44] This study compensated for limitations of previous research both by including a control group and by including a sustained continuous cognitive task. Following baseline self-report measures of fatigue (using the FSS) and depression (using the Center for Epidemiologic Studies-Depression Scale), 59 patients (45 individuals with MS and 14 healthy controls) with varying forms of MS were given a neuropsychological test battery derived from the Brief Repeatable Battery. These included the Selective Reminding Test, the Spatial Recall Test, and the Tower of Hanoi. Patients were then subjected to the Alpha-Arithmetic test, a continuous cognitive effortful task that involves continuous arithmetical calculations, followed by repeat neuropsychological testing.

The MS group exhibited a significant decline in performance on neuropsychological testing following the continuous cognitive task. As seen in Figure 2, the declines were seen on the Selective Reminding Test, indicating decrements in verbal memory.[44]

As with other performance-based studies,[28] the objective changes in cognitive performance did not correlate with self-reported fatigue on the FSS at baseline, nor was there a significant difference in testing outcomes between MS patients with lower FSS scores (<4) versus those with higher scores.

Additional experimental support for cognitive fatigue comes from two separate investigations of MS patients and healthy controls evaluated during a period of sustained performance on a working memory task, the Paced Auditory Serial Addition Test (PASAT). In these studies, MS patients

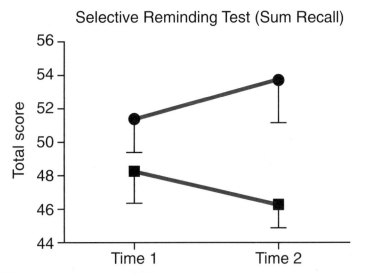

FIGURE 2   Verbal learning before and after a continuous cognitively effortful task in MS and control participants. Circles = control subjects (n=14); squares = patients with MS (n=45). Time 1 indicates battery administered before the continuous cognitively effortful task; time 2 indicates battery administered following the continuous cognitively effortful task. Compared with controls, who improved in the second testing session, a significant decline was seen in the MS patients (*P*=0.035). Adapted from Krupp LB et al. *Neurology.* 2000;55:934–939.[44]

showed declines in performance, defined as an increase in errors over time during a period in which they continuously performed the PASAT. Of note was the finding that even MS patients who appeared relatively cognitively intact compared with controls showed this performance decline over time.[45,46]

Taken together, these studies support the concept of cognitive fatigue. Cognitive fatigue can be best measured by using a continuous cognitive task and by measuring the decrement in performance over time. However, cognitive fatigue is not closely associated with subjective fatigue.

The basis behind cognitive fatigue remains unclear. It may be that the factors such as metabolic dysregulation (e.g., fluctuations in glucose metabolism), which are linked to motor and muscle fatigue, are also responsible for cognitive fatigue. In fact, metabolism in the frontal cortex and basal ganglia, as detected by positron emission tomography (PET) scan, have been associated with higher scores on the FSS in MS patients.[47] Studies conducted using functional MRI in fatigued MS patients performing a simple motor task revealed that those patients with higher reported fatigue on the FSS showed lower activation of cortical and subcortical areas involved in motor planning and execution.[48]

Conclusions

Multiple fatigue assessment instruments are available to measure the patient's level of fatigue. Most are relatively easy to understand, and can be filled out by the patient in the waiting room prior to each visit. Together with the history and physical examination, these measurement scales can be an important tool to assess perceived fatigue severity and distinguish between types of fatigue and its effects on daily activities (physical, cognitive, or psychosocial). Many of the fatigue scales have also shown the ability to demonstrate response to therapy; therefore, they can be used at the time of fatigue diagnosis and periodically thereafter to assess response to therapy. Objective measures of fatigue that assess factors such as muscle strength and recovery time have generally been limited to research applications; however, they may be useful under certain circumstances, as when fatigue is limited to certain muscle groups.

References

1. Freal JE, Kraft GH, Coryell JK. Symptomatic fatigue in multiple sclerosis. *Arch Phys Med Rehabil.* 1984;65:135-138.
2. Multiple Sclerosis Clinical Practice Guidelines: *Fatigue and Multiple Sclerosis: Evidence-Based Management Strategies for Fatigue in Multiple Sclerosis.* Washington, DC: Paralyzed Veterans Association; 1998.
3. Krupp LB, LaRocca NG, Muir-Nash J, Steinberg AD. The Fatigue Severity Scale: application to patients with multiple sclerosis and systemic lupus erythematosus. *Arch Neurol.* 1989;46:1121-1123.
4. Lee KA, Hicks G, Nino-Murcia G. Validity and reliability of a scale to assess fatigue. *Psychiatry Res.* 1991;36:291-298.
5. Borg G. Perceived exertion as an indicator of somatic stress. *Scand J Rehab Med.* 1970;2:92.
6. Borg GA. Psychosocial bases of perceived exertion. *Med Sci Sports Exer.* 1982;14:377-381.
7. Smets EMA, Garssen B, Bonke B, De Haes JCJM. The Multidimensional Fatigue Inventory (MFI): psychometric qualities of an instrument to assess fatigue. *J Psychosom Res.* 1995;39:315-325.
8. Schwartz JE, Jandorf L, Krupp LB. The measurement of fatigue: a new instrument. *J Psychosom Res.* 1993;37:753-762.
9. Stein KD, Martin SC, Hann DM, Jacobsen PB. A multidimensional measure of fatigue for use with cancer patients. *Cancer Pract.* 1998;6:143-152.
10. Fisk JD, Ritvo PG, Ross L, Haase DA, Marrie TJ, Schlech WF. Measuring the functional impact of fatigue: initial validation of the Fatigue Impact Scale. *Clin Infect Dis.* 1994;18:S79-S83.

11. Piper BF, Dibble SL, Dodd MJ, Weiss MC, Slaughter RE, Paul SM. The revised Piper Fatigue Scale: psychometric evaluation in women with breast cancer. *Oncol Nurs Forum.* 1998;25:677-684.

12. Hartz A, Bentler S, Watson D. Measuring fatigue severity in primary care patients. *J Psychosom Res.* 2003;54:515-521.

13. Iriarte J, Katsamakis G, deCastro P. The Fatigue Descriptive Scale (FDS): a useful tool to evaluate fatigue in multiple sclerosis. *Mult Scler.* 1999;5:10-16.

14. Chalder T, Berelowitz G, Pawlikowska T, et al. Development of a Fatigue Scale. *J Psychosom Res.* 1993;37:147-153.

15. Krupp LB, Coyle PK, Doscher C, et al. Fatigue therapy in multiple sclerosis: results of a double-blind, randomized, parallel trial of amantadine, pemoline, and placebo. *Neurology.* 1995;45:1956-1961.

16. Vercoulen JH, Swanink CM, Fennis JF, Galama JM, van der Meer JW, Bleijenberg G. Dimensional assessment of chronic fatigue syndrome. *J Psychosom Res.* 1994;38:383-392.

17. Hann DM, Denniston MM, Baker F. Measurement of fatigue in cancer patients: further validation of the Fatigue Symptom Inventory. *Qual Life Res.* 2000;9: 847-854.

18. Kogi K, Saito Y, Mitsuhashi T. Validity of three components of subjective fatigue feelings. *J Sci Labour.* 1970;46:251-270.

19. Haylock PJ, Hart LK. Fatigue in patients receiving localized radiation. *Cancer Nurs.* 1979;2:461-467.

20. Belza BL. Comparison of self-reported fatigue in rheumatoid arthritis and controls. *J Rheumatol.* 1995;22:639-634.

21. Paul RH, Beatty WW, Schneider R, Blanco CR, Hames KA. Cognitive and physical fatigue in multiple sclerosis: relations between self-report and objective performance. *Appl Neuropsychology.* 1998;5:143-148.

22. Piper BF, Lindsey AM, Dodd MJ, et al. The development of an instrument to measure the subjective dimension of fatigue. In: Funk SG, Tornquist EM, Champagne MT, Copp LA, Wiese RA, eds. *Key Aspects of Comfort: Management of Pain, Fatigue, and Nausea.* New York, NY: Springer Publishing Company; 1989:199-240.

23. Schwid SR, Covington M, Segal BM, Goodman AD. Fatigue in multiple sclerosis: current understanding and future directions. *J Rehab Res Development.* 2002;39:211-224.

24. McNair DM, Lorr M, Droppleman LF. *Profile of Mood States Manual (POMS).* 2nd Ed. San Diego, Calif: Educational and Industrial Testing Service; 1992.

25. Ware JE, Kosinski M, Keller SD. *SF-36 Physical and Mental Health Summary Scales: A User's Manual.* Boston Mass: The Health Institute, New England Medical Center; 1994.

26. Weinshenker BG, Penman M, Bass B, Ebers GC, Rice GPA. A double-blind, randomized crossover trial of pemoline in fatigue associated with multiple sclerosis. *Neurology.* 1992;42:1468-1471.

27. Rammohan KW, Rosenberg JH, Lynn DJ, Blumenfeld AM, Pollack CP, Nagaraja HN. Efficacy and safety of modafinil (Provigil®) for the treatment of fatigue in multiple sclerosis: a two center phase 2 study. *J Neurol Neurosurg Psychiatry.* 2002; 72:179-183.

28. Sheean GL, Murray NMF, Rothwell JC, Miller DH, Thompson AJ. An open-labelled clinical and electrophysiological study of 3,4-diaminopyridine in the treatment of multiple sclerosis. *Brain.* 1998;121:967-975.

29. Taylor RR, Jason LA, Torres A. Fatigue rating scales: an empirical comparison. *Psychol Med.* 2000;30:849-856.

30. LaChapelle DL, Finlayson MA. An evaluation of subjective and objective measures of fatigue in patients with brain injury and healthy controls. *Brain Inj.* 1998;12:649-659.

31. Fisk JD, Pontefract A, Ritvo PG, Archibald CJ, Murray TJ. The impact of fatigue on patients with multiple sclerosis. *Can J Neurol Sci.* 1994;21:9-14.

32. Stone AA, Broderick JE, Porter LS, et al. Fatigue and mood in chronic fatigue syndrome patients: results of a momentary assessment protocol examining fatigue and mood levels and diurnal patterns. *Ann Behav Med.* 1994;16:228-234.

33. Meek PM, Nail LM, Barsevick A, et al. Psychometric testing of fatigue instruments for use with cancer patients. *Nurs Res.* 2000;49:181-190.

34. Djaldetti R, Zif I, Achiron A, Melamed E. Fatigue in multiple sclerosis compared with chronic fatigue syndrome: a quantitative assessment. *Neurology.* 1996;46:632-635.

35. deHaan A, deRuiter CJ, van der Woude LHV, Jongen PJH. Contractile properties and fatigue of quadriceps muscles in multiple sclerosis. *Musc Nerve.* 2000;23:1534-1541.

36. Petajan JH, White AT. Motor-evoked potentials in response to fatiguing grip exercise in multiple sclerosis patients. *Clin Neurophysiol.* 2000;111:2188-2195.

37. Monks J. Experiencing symptoms in chronic illness: fatigue in multiple sclerosis. *Int Disabil Study.* 1989;11:78-83.

38. Rao S, Leo G, Ellington L, et al. Cognitive function in multiple sclerosis, II: impact on employment social functioning. *Neurology.* 1991;41:692-696.

39. Schwartz CE, Coulthard-Morris L, Zeng Q. Psychosocial correlates of fatigue in multiple sclerosis. *Arch Phys Med Rehabil.* 1996;77:165-170.

40. Parmenter BA, Denney DR, Lynch SG. The cognitive performance of patients with multiple sclerosis during periods of high and low fatigue. *Mult Scler.* 2003;9:111-118.

41. Geisler MW, Sliwinski M, Coyle PK, Masur DM, Doscher C, Krupp LB. The effects of amantadine and pemoline on cognitive functioning in multiple sclerosis. *Arch Neurol.* 1996;53:185-188.

42. Caruso L, LaRocca N, Foley F, et al. Exertional fatigue fails to affect cognitive function in multiple sclerosis. *J Clin Exp Neuropsychol.* 1991;13:74. Abstract.

43. Kujala P, Portin R, Reconsuo A, Ruutiainen J. Attention related performance in two cognitively different subgroups of patients with multiple sclerosis. *J Neurol Neurosurg Psychiatry.* 1995;59:77-82.

44. Krupp LB, Elkins LE. Fatigue and declines in cognitive functioning in multiple sclerosis. *Neurology.* 2000;55:934-939.

45. Bryant D, Chiaravalloti ND, DeLuca J. Objective measures of cognitive fatigue in multiple sclerosis. *Rehabil Psychology.* 2004. In press.

46. Schwid SR, Tyler CM, Scheid EA, Weinstein A, Goodman AD, McDermott MLP. Cognitive fatigue during a test requiring sustained attention: a pilot study. *Mult Scler.* 2003;9:503-508.

47. Roelcke U, Kappos L, Lechner-Scott J, Brunnschweiler H, Huber S, Ammann W. Reduced glucose metabolism in the frontal cortex and basal ganglia of multiple sclerosis patients with fatigue: an ^{18}F-fluorodeoxyglucose positron emission tomography study. *Neurology.* 1997;48:1566-1571.

48. Filippi M, Rocca MA, Colombo B, et al. Functional magnetic resonance imaging correlates of fatigue in multiple sclerosis. *Neuroimage.* 2002;15:559-567.

CHAPTER 4
Pathophysiology

Why do people with MS experience fatigue? A complete physiologic explanation for MS fatigue is beyond our current level of knowledge of the central nervous system (CNS) or of MS. Nonetheless, there has been considerable effort towards explaining this symptom. The major proposed pathophysiologic mechanisms for fatigue can be categorized according to: 1) the autoimmune nature of MS and its associated disrupted immune responses; 2) the impaired neuronal functioning caused by CNS demyelination and axonal destruction; and 3) alterations in neuroendocrine feedback. Additional proposed mechanisms that have been studied as explanations for MS fatigue are autonomic nervous system dysregulation and deficits related to energy conservation. These different mechanisms likely interact with one another, with no one pathway serving as the sole cause for MS fatigue.

Definition of Fatigue and Explanations

Explanations for fatigue vary on which definition of the symptom is being considered. In this chapter, the sense of exhaustion reported by individuals with MS as one of their primary concerns is the phenomenon we are trying to explain. Fatigue in this sense is not adequately accounted for by gender, psychosomatic mechanisms, motor impairments, or sleep dysfunction. Large demographic studies have shown either weak or minimal correlation with age or disease duration.[1]

The physiologic definition of fatigue as performance decrement is a useful descriptive term, but does not provide a pathophysiologic mechanism for perceived states of exhaustion because most motor or cognitive measures are not meaningfully associated with perceived fatigue.[2-4] In contrast, studies of perceived fatigue measured by self-report scales have led to some supportive experimental data regarding brain metabolism and fatigue, and have allowed inferences of MS fatigue to be drawn from other medical disorders.

Proposed Mechanisms of MS-Related Fatigue

Immune Dysregulation and Fatigue

There is strong evidence that alterations in immune system activity play a substantial role in fatigue in the MS patient. Fatigue is a significant symptom across several autoimmune disorders aside from MS, including systemic lupus erythematosus (SLE).[5] In the cases of both MS and SLE, fatigue can be the first symptom of an impending relapse or flare.

In chronic fatigue syndrome (CFS), where fatigue is the essence of the condition, there are several changes consistent with decreased cellular immunity that have been reported, including increases in the number of activated T lymphocytes and inflammatory cytokines such as interleukin-1 (IL-1) and tumor necrosis factor-alpha (TNF-alpha).[6] It has been suggested that these cytokines may accumulate during periods of wakefulness and thereby promote daytime fatigue.[6]

Immune activation may exert effects on fatigue in the MS patient through changes in neuroendocrine function, by promoting the secretion of corticotropin-releasing hormone (CRH), adrenocorticotropic hormone (ACTH), and cortisol.[6] An association has also been proposed between fatigue and thyroid function,[7] with a case study in a patient with MS-related fatigue showing the presence of autoimmune thyroid disease following interferon-beta administration.[8] Hence, interaction with thyroid function may underlie the fatigue associated with interferon immune modulating therapies.

Attempts to correlate MS fatigue with circulating levels of cytokines have been inconsistent. Multiple sclerosis is associated with increased changes in CD4 cell subsets, which lead to elevations in proinflammatory cytokines.[9] Changes in both proinflammatory and anti-inflammatory cytokines have been associated with fatigue. In at least one study of MS patients, levels of circulating cytokines were linked to fatigue.[10] However, these findings have not been replicated by other groups.[11] Given the sensitivity of circulating inflammatory cytokines to so many variables and the multiple factors affecting measurement of cytokine levels, it is not surprising that associations between circulating levels of cytokines and other biologic markers of immune activity and fatigue would be difficult to detect. Evidence for an association between fatigue and various CD receptor T cell subsets and cytokines such as IL-1, IL-6, and TNF-alpha in patients with CFS has also been inconsistent.

Another line of evidence for a role of immune system dysregulation in producing fatigue relates to how the class of immune modulators, the interferon betas, clearly produces fatigue as a side effect. The interferons have been associated with the induction of a flu-like reaction that includes fatigue, fever, and chills, not only in MS but in other disorders such as cancer.[12-14] The precise mechanism by which the interferon betas induce fatigue is unclear. In one study of healthy individuals, interferon beta administration was associated with an increase in inflammatory cytokine levels, including TNF-alpha, IL-1, and IL-6.[15] In contrast, another study of healthy volunteers found that interferon beta administration resulted in decreases in the levels of cytokines, though fatigue was still a prominent side effect.[16]

Whatever the precise mechanism, fatigue or a "flu-like symptom complex" has been reported in 41% to 76% of patients in the phase 3 clinical MS trials of the interferon betas.[17-19] This type of reaction was considerably lower (approximately 19%) in the phase 3 trials of glatiramer acetate, which is not a naturally occurring protein but a synthetic preparation that has immune-modifying properties.[20] The mechanism of action of glatiramer acetate is sufficiently distinct from the mechanism of action of the interferon betas that it is not surprising that the side-effect profile is quite different.[21]

Potential differences between the interferon betas and glatiramer acetate relative to fatigue symptoms were noted in a study that used the Fatigue Impact Scale (FIS, see Chapter 3) to assess fatigue symptoms in patients taking any of the four available disease-modifying therapies for at least 6 months. Compared with baseline FIS assessments, 25% of individuals taking glatiramer acetate showed reductions (i.e., improvement) in FIS scores, compared with 12% of those taking any of the interferon betas ($P=0.02$). The reduction in the fatigue was seen on all three of the subscales of the FIS: physical functioning, cognitive functioning, and social functioning, and the odds ratio for having an improved FIS score was 2.2 for glatiramer acetate compared with the interferon betas.[22]

Two other studies have also shown positive symptomatic effects relative to glatiramer acetate in MS patients. One identified positive effects of the medication on upper and lower extremity muscle strength in 64 patients before and after the initiation of glatiramer acetate therapy.[23]

Another investigation of MS patients found that those who performed a physically fatiguing task while on one of the interferon betas had a significantly greater postural tremor amplitude ($P=0.015$) compared with those on glatiramer acetate.[24]

In severely fatigued patients, the side-effect profile with the disease-modifying therapies is an issue to consider in choosing a particular therapy. This is especially important, as interferon-related fatigue can have an effect on adherence to therapy. In an open-label trial of 72 patients who received interferon beta-1b, a number of side effects, including fatigue, depression, and headache, were observed. However, fatigue and a "fatigue-depression interaction" were the only symptoms significantly predictive of therapy discontinuation.[12,14]

It is clear that medications and other factors affecting immune function may contribute to fatigue. However, immune dysfunction is only one underlying mechanism for fatigue, and many other causes also contribute to the phenomenon. Since fatigue occurs during relapse-free periods and in progressive forms of MS that are considered less likely to be as inflammatory, it is reasonable to conclude that CNS mechanisms also play a key role.

Central Nervous System Mechanisms

Several distinct areas of the CNS are believed to be involved in the pathophysiology of MS-related fatigue, including the premotor cortex, the limbic system, the basal ganglia, and the brain-stem. Hypofunctioning in these areas could lead to decreased motor readiness, resulting in fatigue. The dysfunction in these CNS regions could result from immune injury, neuronal dysfunction secondary to demyelination of nerve sheaths and destruction of axons, and other changes resulting from a state of recurrent or chronic CNS inflammation.

Functional imaging studies, including functional MRI (fMRI) and positron emission tomography (PET), have yielded provocative findings that may be relative to the study of MS fatigue. In one fMRI study, significantly lower activation of several brain areas involved in motor planning and execution, including the thalamus, was seen in MS patients.[25] This is important, as the thalamus is an important relay station that links the motor and prefrontal cortices to the basal ganglia, and is part of the feedback loops of the limbic system that serve to modulate cortical motor output.[25,26] Reduced activation of select areas including the contralateral thalamus, was associated with higher fatigue scores on the FSS.[25] Other studies employing PET imaging have demonstrated significant hypometabolism in the prefrontal cortex and basal ganglia of MS patients, with mean reductions in total brain glucose metabolism of approximately 10% to 20% compared with normal individuals.[27,28] Decreased glucose metabolism was demonstrated in the MS patients with fatigue in one of these studies.[28]

Reduced frontal lobe activity has also been associated with fatigue in other progressive CNS disorders, such as Parkinson's disease.[29] Parallel findings such as these in other neurodegenerative disorders lend support to the importance of CNS perfusion deficits and decreased glucose uptake in fatigue pathophysiology.

While efforts that tie neuronal function to fatigue have met with some success, investigations attempting to identify a specific neuroanatomic locus for fatigue have not been as promising. Several MRI studies have failed to establish an association between MS fatigue and lesion load or brain atrophy.[30,31] Given the complex and multifaceted nature of fatigue, it seems less likely that one brain location would correlate with this symptom.

The way in which demyelination in MS contributes to fatigue is not clear, but has been the subject of much speculation and research. It has been suggested that impaired innervation of muscle groups may require a compensatory increase in central motor drive exertion,[32] causing the individual to expend a greater degree of energy for a given level of motor function. In support of this, studies employing quantitative measures of electromyography and voluntary muscle contraction have attributed decreases in muscle force generation to changes in central motor drive.[33,34] The resulting muscle fatigue as a result of these impairments has been distinguished from muscle "weakness."[35] However, a limitation of research into a CNS mechanism for fatigue has been the poor correlation between self-reported fatigue and changes in central motor activation or muscle activation.[33]

Perhaps one of the factors most characteristic of fatigue in MS that is not seen in other disease states is the strong association between heat and fatigue. Excessive heating in the MS patient exacerbates fatigue, perhaps through disrupted conduction that requires an increase in heat-generating exertion to achieve a given level of physical activity.[32] The sensitivity of MS fatigue to heat is likely a consequence of the CNS nature of the symptom.

The importance of cerebral mechanisms in fatigue is supported at least in part by the apparent correlation between fatigue and depression. A significant relationship between fatigue and depression in MS was noted in a study of 71 patients, with depressed patients having higher FSS scores than nondepressed patients, even after controlling for physical disability.[36] It has been proposed that the correlation between depression and fatigue, independent of the level of physical disability, suggests that dysfunction along specific neural pathways may play a role in both MS-related fatigue and depression.[36]

Neuroendocrine/Neurotransmitter Dysregulation

As noted above, it is likely that endocrinal abnormalities, such as abnormal thyroid functioning, play at least a partial role in fatigue development.[8] Most research in this area, however, has focused on the role of the hypothalamic-pituitary-adrenal (HPA) axis (Figure 1), which is the body's stress regulator.[37]

Support for a significant role of the HPA axis in fatigue pathophysiology is found in CFS and fibromyalgia. Reduced activation of the adrenal

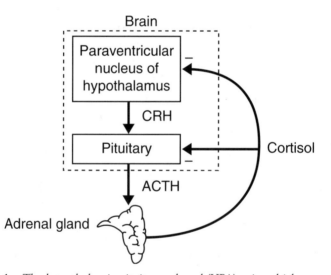

FIGURE 1   The hypothalamic-pituitary-adrenal (HPA) axis, which serves as the body's stress regulator. In response to stress, the hypothalamus releases corticotropin-releasing hormone (CRH), which triggers the release of adrenocorticotropic hormone (ACTH) from the pituitary gland. ACTH acts on the adrenal cortex, causing it to release cortisol in the bloodstream. Cortisol exerts a "negative feedback" effect on the hypothalamus to inhibit further CRH release and thus reduce cortisol levels. A condition of chronic stress can result in prolonged depletion of cortisol levels, potentially leading to fatigue. One interesting study demonstrated that interferon beta-1b exerts a stimulatory effect on the HPA axis that may contribute to side effects.

gland, with low circulating levels of the stress hormone cortisol, in response to physical and emotional stressors, may underlie the physiologic changes associated with CFS, and may account for the severe fatigue.[38,39] It is possible that the HPA axis may exert a similar influence in MS fatigue.

Several studies have been specifically performed on HPA axis dysregulation in MS patients. One group studied HPA axis activity in 52 patients with clinically definite MS, concluding that activation of the HPA axis occurs secondary to active inflammation.[40] Administration of interferon beta to healthy subjects leads to significant increases in proinflammatory cytokines, as well as elevations in cortisol, prolactin, and growth hormone plasma levels. The link between cytokines, interferon beta, and the HPA axis may underlie the fatigue associated with interferon beta administration in the MS patient. One interesting study demonstrated that interferon beta-1b exerts a stimulatory effect on the HPA axis that may contribute to fatigue side effects.[15]

While HPA axis dysregulation appears to play some causative role in the development of fatigue, it remains unclear whether endocrine dysfunction is a primary or secondary cause of fatigue. For example it is possible that a reduction in cortisol levels occurs secondary to changes in sleep or exercise. It has been observed that changes in cortisol levels are often not exceptional enough to account for the significant fatigue associated with CFS.[6]

The hypothalamus, and pathways involving neurotransmitters such as dopamine, histamine, and serotonin, are also likely to contribute to fatigue pathogenesis. For example, it has been argued that disruption in serotonergic pathways interferes with attention, and could lead to cognitive fatigue.[41,42] Effects on the hypothalamus can lead to decreased arousal and hence, increased fatigue. The observation that modafinil reduces fatigue in MS, and is a medication that is hypothesized to exert its effects via nondopaminergic mechanisms mediated through the hypothalamus, provides indirect evidence of the importance of hypothalamic mechanisms in fatigue.[43,44] It may also be that fatigue as a symptom depends on defects in both neuroendocrine and neurotransmitter systems, as well as the interactions between these systems and the hypothalamus.

Autonomic Nervous System Involvement

Other pathophysiologic bases for fatigue have been explored in patients with chronic disease, including those with MS. It has been theorized that clinical symptoms of cardiovascular autonomic dysregulation (e.g., dizziness, weakness, neurocognitive complaints, and exhaustion) are similar to symptoms reported by those with fatigue. In a study of 84 MS patients, 64% of whom were fatigued, approximately 20% had coexistent signs of autonomic failure and fatigue.[45] In a study of autonomic tests and measures of heart rate variability in 60 MS patients, an association was seen between fatigue and hypoadrenergic orthostatic response, which was interpreted as due to impaired sympathetic vasomotor function with intact vagal heart control.[46] However, in other studies of autonomic function in which autonomic instability has been measured by pupillary unrest,[47] there was no positive correlation seen with fatigue severity. Taken together, these data show a need for additional investigation before a conclusion regarding the influence of autonomic dysregulation and fatigue in MS can be drawn.

Energy Depletion

Fatigue has been linked to energy depletion in a number of conditions, both chronic (e.g., cancer) and acute (e.g., the postsurgical state).[6,48] Although the issue of fatigue and energy depletion due to chronic illness has not been researched directly in the MS patient, it is likely that the extreme metabolic demands placed on the body in battling a chronic illness such as MS may contribute to a fatigued state.

Fatigue Cofactors

There are a number of factors that, while not considered causes of primary MS-related fatigue, may serve as secondary contributors. These include affective/mood disorders (discussed in Chapter 5), pain, deconditioning, sleep disorders, and medications used to treat other symptoms of MS. As with primary causes of MS-related fatigue, these cofactors can overlap and exacerbate each other, increasing the severity of existing fatigue. For example, the use of sedatives or muscle relaxants can decrease daytime energy and interfere with muscle functioning, leading to decreases in exercise. This, in turn, increases deconditioning and symptoms of fatigue.

Sleep Dysfunction

Nighttime sleep disruption often contributes to daytime symptoms of fatigue, in MS as well as other fatiguing disorders.[49] Sleep disorders are common among the general population (with an estimated prevalence of 12%),[50] and have been estimated to be up to three times more common in MS patients.[51] In the MS patient, motor problems such as nocturnal spasms or spasticity are the most common causes of disruption of night-time sleep duration or quality. In addition, nocturia and incontinence can frequently interrupt sleep patterns and lead to daytime fatigue. Finally, MS patients are susceptible to unrelated conditions such as obstructive sleep apnea hypopnea syndrome.

It is important to try to determine the basis for reports of sleepiness in the fatigued patient. Often, the patient's bed partner is the most valuable resource for diagnosing a sleep disorder. The physician should query the patient's bed partner about the presence of disrupted sleep pattern or apneas/hypopneas. Subjective sleep questionnaires such as the Epworth Sleepiness Scale can be used to diagnose the presence and severity of sleepiness symptoms, and to assess response to interventions such as stimulant medications or modafinil.

Some researchers have reported an association between MS and primary sleep disorders, such as REM-sleep behavior disorder.[52] On occasion, patients may complain of severely disrupted sleep or sudden sleep episodes that intrude into normal wakefulness, which may indicate a primary sleep disorder such as narcolepsy.[53] In such cases, referral to a sleep clinic for polysomnographic monitoring may be indicated to diagnose a primary sleep disorder. Given the potential severe consequences of obstructive sleep apnea hypopnea syndrome, including hypertension and cardiovascular disease,[54] patients with this condition should also be referred to a sleep disorders specialist for appropriate treatment.

Pain

Pain and fatigue often overlap, and both can have a substantial detrimental impact on functioning.[6] Sensory disturbances including neuralgia, dysesthesia, and paroxysmal painful spasms all occur in individuals with MS.[55,56] Pain can contribute to fatigue by limiting activity, thereby increasing physical deconditioning. The presence of nighttime pain can interfere with normal sleep and cause daytime fatigue and/or sleepiness. Pain can also contribute to depression, which may be closely associated with fatigue.[57] In addition, it is likely that the experience of moving and functioning in pain is energy consuming, and leads to a depletion of reserves.

As in fatigue or sleepiness, self-report scales, such as the Visual Analog Scale, can be used to assess the patient's level of pain. Pain due to spasticity should be treated appropriately with analgesics and antispasticity medications (e.g., tizanidine or baclofen). In patients who report that they are severely disabled by pain, a multidisciplinary approach that considers mechanisms of coping, contribution of affective disorders, and psychosocial support should be included in addition to pharmacologic or physical therapy interventions.

Physical Deconditioning

Deconditioning from failure or an inability to exercise can exacerbate fatigue in MS. Patients who exhibit increasing levels of weakness as the disease progresses may experience a decrease in aerobic capacity. Individuals with fatigue may avoid activities such as exercise, which is a problem, as lack of excercise can worsen fatigue over the long term. In persons who are severely disabled and unable to move, the respiratory muscles can become weakened, causing the body to use increasing amounts of energy to breathe.[58,59] Exercise/reconditioning programs are a treatment strategy that must be prescribed within the physical limitations of the individual (see Chapter 7).

Medication Use

Medications used to treat other symptoms of MS, such as spasticity and pain, often have side effects that include fatigue. Among the most common classes of medications associated with fatiguing side effects are analgesics (e.g., opioids), antispasticity agents (e.g., tizanidine and baclofen), sedatives and antihypnotics (e.g., diazepam or zolpidem), anticonvulsants (e.g., carbamazepine), and antihistamines (e.g., diphenhydramine). An inclusive list of potentially fatiguing medications that are often used in the MS patient can be found in the guidelines on fatigue promulgated by the MS Council for Clinical Practice Guidelines.[60] The guidelines can be obtained by contacting the Paralyzed Veterans Association or visiting its website at www.pva.org. (A comprehensive list is also found in Chapter 8.)

As noted above, in addition to the medications used for symptom management, the interferon betas have been associated with fatiguing side effects. The fatigue that occurs with interferon beta therapy generally is part of a postinjection, flu-like reaction that also includes fever and chills. This reaction generally subsides over time.

Conclusions

The pathophysiologic underpinnings of MS-related fatigue are multifactorial. Fatigue in the MS patient most likely appears to be the result of alterations in immune system function, functional consequences of pathologic changes in the nervous system related to the disease process, and neuroendocrine changes. Numerous other disease features, including sleep dysregulation, pain, chronic illness factors, psychologic factors, and deconditioning. However, none of these features alone fully accounts for the fatigue experienced by the MS patient. Fatigue remains an enigma; however, continued progress in defining its pathophysiology will undoubtedly lead to improvements in therapy.

References

1. Lerdal A, Celius EG, Moum T. Fatigue and its association with sociodemographic variables among multiple sclerosis patients. *Mult Scler.* 2003;9:509-514.
2. Krupp LB, Elkins LE. Fatigue and declines in cognitive functioning in multiple sclerosis. *Neurology.* 2000;55:934-939.
3. Sharma KR, Kent-Braun J, Mynhier MA, Weiner MW, Miller RG. Evidence of an abnormal intramuscular component of fatigue in multiple sclerosis. *Muscle Nerve.* 1995;18:1403-1411.
4. Parmenter BA, Denney DR, Lynch SG. The cognitive performance of patients with multiple sclerosis during periods of high and low fatigue. *Mult Scler.* 2003;9:111-118.
5. Krupp LB, LaRocca NG, Muir J, Steinberg AD. Fatigue characteristics in systemic lupus erythematosus. *J Rheumatol.* 1990;17:1450-1452.
6. Wessely S, Hotopf M, Sharpe M. *Chronic Fatigue and its Syndromes.* London, UK: Oxford University Press; 1999.
7. Jones TH, Wadler S, Hupart KH. Endocrine-mediated mechanisms of fatigue during treatment with interferon-alpha. *Semin Oncol.* 1998;25(suppl 1):54-63.
8. Schwid SR, Goodman AD, Mattson DH. Autoimmune hyperthyroidism in patients with multiple sclerosis treated with interferon beta-1b. *Arch Neurol.* 1997;57:1169-1170.
9. Hemmer B, Cepok S, Nessler S, Sommer N. Pathogenesis of multiple sclerosis: an update on immunology. *Curr Opin Neurol.* 2002;15:227-231.
10. Iriarte J, Subira ML, Castro P. Modalities of fatigue in multiple sclerosis: correlation with clinical and biological factors. *Mult Scler.* 2000;6:124-130.
11. Giovannoni G, Thompson AJ, Miller DH, Thompson EJ. Fatigue is not associated with raised inflammatory markers in multiple sclerosis. *Neurology.* 2001;57:676-681.
12. Neilly LK, Goodin DS, Goodkin DE, Hause SL. Side effect profile of interferon beta-1b in MS: results of an open label trial. *Neurology.* 1996;46:552-554.
13. Quesada JR, Talpax M, Rios A, et al. Clinical toxicity of interferons in cancer patients: a review. *J Clin Oncol.* 1986;4:234-243.
14. Gottberg K, Gardulf A, Fredrikson S. Interferon-beta treatment for patients with multiple sclerosis: the patients' perceptions of side effects. *Mult Scler.* 2000;6:349-354.
15. Goebel M, Basse J, Pithan V, et al. Acute interferon beta-1b administration alters hypothalamic-pituitary-adrenal axis activity, plasma cytokines and leukocyte distribution in healthy subjects. *Psychoneuroendocrinology.* 2002;27:881.
16. Rothuizen L, Buclin T, Spertini F, et al. Influence of interferon b-1a dose frequency on PBMC cytokine secretion and biological effect markers. *J Neuroimmunol.* 1999;99:131-141.

17. Avonex® (Interferon beta-1a) prescribing information. Cambridge, Mass: Biogen, Inc.; 2003.

18. Betaseron® (interferon beta-1b) prescribing information. Richmond, Calif; Berlex Laboratories; 2002.

19. Rebif® (Interferon beta-1a) prescribing information. Rockland, MA; Serono, Inc.; 2003.

20. Copaxone® (Glatiramer acetate) prescribing information. Kansas City, MO: Teva; 2003.

21. Chabot S, Yong FP, Le DM, Metz LM, Myles T, Yong VW. Cytokine production in T lymphocyte-microglia interaction is attenuated by glatiramer acetate: a mechanism for therapeutic efficacy in multiple sclerosis. *Mult Scler.* 2002;8:299-306.

22. Metz LM, Patten SB, Rose SM, et al. Multiple sclerosis fatigue is decreased at 6 months by glatiramer acetate (Copaxone). *J Neurol.* 2001;248(suppl 2):115.

23. Sanjak M, Yenter K, Belden DS, Konopacki RA, Brooks BR. Glatiramer acetate [GA] treatment effects on computerized isometric muscle strength [CIMS] in multiple sclerosis [MS] patients: a longitudinal MS clinic-based study. Presented at: the 18th Congress of the European Committee for Research and Treatment in Multiple Sclerosis (ECTRIMS). Baltimore, MD; September 20, 2001. Abstract P195.

24. Dogan S, Konopacki RA, Sanjak M, et al. Glatiramer acetate [GA] treatment effects on fatigue-induced tremor amplitude in multiple sclerosis [MS] patients. Presented at: the 18th Congress of the European Committee for Research and Treatment in Multiple Sclerosis (ECTRIMS). Baltimore, MD; September 20, 2001. Abstract P188.

25. Filippi M, Rocca MA, Colombo B, et al. Functional magnetic resonance imaging correlates of fatigue in multiple sclerosis. *Neuroimage.* 2002;15:559-567.

26. Chaudhuri A, Behan PO. Fatigue and basal ganglia. *J Neurol Sci.* 2000;179:34-42.

27. Bakshi R, Miletich RS, Kinkel PR, et al. High-resolution fluorodeoxyglucose positron emission tomography shows both global and regional cerebral hypometabolism in multiple sclerosis. *J Neuroimaging.* 1998;8:228-234.

28. Roelcke U, Kappos L, Lechner-Scott, et al. Reduced glucose metabolism in the frontal cortex and basal ganglia of multiple sclerosis patients with fatigue: an 18F-fluorodeoxyglucose positron emission tomography study. *Neurology.* 1997;48:1566-1571.

29. Abe K, Takanashi M, Yanagihara T. Fatigue in patients with Parkinson's disease. *Behav Neurol.* 2000;12:103-106.

30. Mainero C, Faroni J, Gasperini C, et al. Fatigue and magnetic resonance imaging activity in multiple sclerosis. *J Neurol.* 1999;246:454-458.

31. Bakshi R, Miletich R, Henschel K, et al. Fatigue in multiple sclerosis: cross-sectional correlation with brain MRI findings in 71 patients. *Neurology.* 1999;53:1151-1153.

32. Bakshi R. Fatigue associated with multiple sclerosis: diagnosis, impact and management. *Mult Scler.* 2003;9:219-227.

33. Sheean GL, Murray NMF, Rothwell C, et al. An electrophysiological study of the mechanism of fatigue in multiple sclerosis. *Brain.* 1997;120(suppl 2):299-315.

34. Ng AV, Miller RG, Kent-Braun JA. Central motor drive is increased during voluntary muscle contractions in multiple sclerosis. *Musc Nerve.* 1997;20:1213-1218.

35. Schwid SR, Thorton CA, Pandya S, et al. Quantitative assessment of motor fatigue and strength in MS. *Neurology.* 1999;53:743-750.

36. Bakshi R, Shaikh ZA, Miletich RS, et al. Fatigue in multiple sclerosis and its relationship to depression and neurologic disability. *Mult Scler.* 2000;6:181-185.
37. Krupp LB. *Fatigue: The Most Common Complaints.* Philadelphia, PA: Elsevier Science; 2003.
38. Demitrack MA, Crofford LJ. Evidence for and pathophysiologic implications of hypothalamic-pituitary-adrenal axis dysregulation in fibromyalgia and chronic fatigue syndrome. *Ann N Y Acad Sci.* 1998;840-684-697.
39. Ehlert U, Gaab J, Henrichs M. Psychoneuroendocrinological contributions to the etiology of depression, posttraumatic stress disorder, and stress-related bodily disorders: the role of the hypothalamus-pituitary-adrenal axis. *Biol Psychiatry.* 2001;57:141-152.
40. Wei T, Lightman SL. The neuroendocrine axis in patients with multiple sclerosis. *Brain.* 1997;120:1067-1076.
41. Parker AJ, Wessely S, Cleare AJ. The neuroendocrinology of chronic fatigue syndrome and fibromyalgia. *Psychol Med.* 2001;31:1331-1345.
42. Heilman KM, Watson RT. Fatigue. *Neurology Network Commentary.* 1997;1:283-287.
43. Scammell TE, Estabrooke IV, McCarthy MT, et al. Hypothalamic arousal regions are activated during modafinil-induced wakefulness. *J Neurosci.* 2000;20:8620-8628.
44. Rammohan KW, Rosenberg JH, Lynn DJ, Blumenfeld AM, Pollak CP, Nagaraja HN. Efficacy and safety of modafinil (Provigil®) for the treatment of fatigue in multiple sclerosis: a two centre phase 2 study. *J Neurol Neurosurg Psychiatry.* 2002;72:179-183.
45. Merkelbach S, Dillman U, Kolmel C, Holz J, Muller M. Cardiovascular autonomic dysregulation and fatigue in multiple sclerosis. *Mult Scler.* 2001;7:320-326.
46. Flachenecker P, Rufer A, Bihler I, et al. Fatigue in MS is related to sympathetic vasomotor dysfunction. *Neurology.* 2003;61:851-853.
47. Egg R, Hogl B, Glatzl S, Beer R, Berger T. Autonomic instability, as measured by pupillary unrest, is not associated with multiple sclerosis fatigue severity. *Mult Scler.* 2002;8:256-260.
48. Holley S. Cancer-related fatigue: suffering a different fatigue. *Cancer Pract.* 2000;8:87-95.
49. Morrison RE, Keating HJ. Fatigue in primary care. *Obstet Gynecol Clin North Am.* 2001;28:225-237.
50. Happe S. Excessive daytime sleepiness and sleep disturbances in patients with neurological diseases: epidemiology and management. *Drugs.* 2003;63:2725-2737.
51. Clark CM, Fleming JA, Li D, Oger J, Klonoff H, Paty D. Sleep disturbance, depression, and lesion site in patients with multiple sclerosis. *Arch Neurol.* 1992;49:641-643.
52. Ferini-Strambi L, Zucconi M. REM sleep behavior disorder. *Clin Neurophysiol.* 2000;111(Suppl 2):S136-S140.
53. American Sleep Disorders Association: *The International Classification of Sleep Disorders: Diagnostic and Coding Manual.* Revised. Rochester, Minnesota: American Sleep Disorders Association; 1997.
54. Attarian HP, Sabri AN. When to suspect obstructive sleep apnea syndrome: symptoms may be subtle, but straightforward. *Postgrad Med.* 2002;111:70-76.
55. Schapiro RT. Pharmacologic options for the management of multiple sclerosis symptoms. *Neurorehabil Neural Repair.* 2002;16:223-231.
56. Stenager E, Knudsen L, Jensen K. Acute and chronic pain syndromes in multiple sclerosis. *Acta Neurol Scand.* 1991;84:197-200.

57. Flachenecker P, Kumpfel T, Kallmann B, et al. Fatigue in multiple sclerosis: a comparison of different rating scales and correlation to clinical parameters. *Mult Scler.* 2002;8:523-526.

58. Foglio K, Clini E, Facchetti D. Respiratory muscle function and exercise capacity in MS. *Eur Resp J.* 1994;7:23-28.

59. Smeltzer SC, Lavietes MH, Cook SD. Expiratory training in multiple sclerosis. *Arch Phys Med Rehabil* 1996;77:909-912.

60. Multiple Sclerosis Clinical Practice Guidelines: *Fatigue and Multiple Sclerosis: Evidence-Based Management Strategies for Fatigue in Multiple Sclerosis.* Washington, DC: Paralyzed Veterans Association, 1998.

CHAPTER 5

Depression/Affective State and Its Relationship to MS-Related Fatigue

Fatigue and affect often show a reciprocal interaction in chronic medical disorders. In multiple sclerosis (MS), in particular, it is clear that depression, coping style, personality traits, and each individual's interpretation of the disease influences the experience of fatigue. This chapter reviews the relationships between fatigue, mood, and psychologic consequences of MS in greater detail.

Depression and Fatigue

The most notable affective disorder associated with MS is depression. Over 50% of MS patients will have a diagnosable depressive disorder over the course of their lifetime,[1] and the point prevalence of significant depressive symptoms is also very high.[2] The unpredictable nature of MS and its severe disabling symptoms (including fatigue) contribute to mood disorders. However, depression appears to be more common in MS compared with other similarly disabling neurologic disorders.[3] Depressive symptoms occur in patients with all stages of MS, including those with a recent diagnosis, as well as those with greater levels of neurologic impairment.[4]

The higher frequency of depression in MS has been explained by pathologic and immune consequences of the disease, including damage to different regions of the brain. Lesion burden in the frontal lobes, periventricular region, and temporal lobes correlates positively with depressive symptoms in MS in some, but not all, neuroimaging studies.[3]

Symptoms of depression aggravate fatigue, either directly or through other psychologic consequences.[5–7] Depression may add to the deficits in executive functioning that are already often present in MS.[8] Depression can also lead to somatization disorder in chronic illness, which increases the severity of disability associated with a given level of neurologic impairment.[9] The stresses associated with chronic illness can increase the severity of depressive symptoms. In addition, physical impairments and fatigue can affect depression through an association with decreased recreational activity.[10] It is possible that decreased recreational functioning can in turn lead to greater social isolation and further deconditioning, which can further add to fatigue.

Fatigue, neurologic impairment as measured by the EDSS, and depression are also inter-related.[11–14] However, in at least one study, once depression was controlled for the association between fatigue and neurologic impairment was very much attenuated.[11]

Depression in association with severe chronic fatigue has been linked to changes in neurohormonal or immunologic function. A growing body of research supports a relationship between stressful life events and psychologic distress, and impairments in cellular immunity.[9] It is reasonable to assume that these stress-related factors can further add to the fatigue of MS.

It is critical to evaluate MS patients for the presence of symptoms of depression and treat these symptoms aggressively (Table 1).[15] Treating depression through either cognitive-behavioral therapy or antidepressant medication lowers fatigue levels in depressed MS patients,[16] as well as in other fatigue states such as chronic fatigue syndrome.[17] Depression treatment should precede or occur simultaneously with other strategies for reducing fatigue.

Fatigue and mood both vary over time, and can be affected by different factors in the disease course. Examining fatigue as a multidimensional phenomenon has shown that mental fatigue and physical fatigue may correlate differently with depression when assessed in a cross-sectional versus a longitudinal analysis. In a study of 98 MS patients evaluated at baseline and over one year, depression was significantly correlated at baseline with mental fatigue but one year later was predictive of only physical fatigue. Hence the relationships over time between mood and different fatigue dimensions are complex.[18] In contrast, a study using a unidimensional measure of fatigue, in which changes in fatigue and depression were measured over the course of a clinical trial, showed a relative independence between fatigue and mood.[19]

TABLE 1 *DSM-IV* Diagnostic Criteria for Depression

Major Depressive Episode*:

A. Five (or more) of the following symptoms have been present during the same two-week period and represent a change from previous functioning; at least one of the symptoms is either: 1) depressed mood, or 2) loss of interest or pleasure. (Do not include symptoms that are clearly due to a general medical condition, or mood-incongruent delusions or hallucinations.)

   1. Depressed mood most of the day, nearly every day, as indicated by either subjective report (e.g., feels sad or empty) or observation made by others (e.g., appears tearful).

   2. Markedly diminished interest or pleasure in all, or almost all, activities most of the day, nearly every day (as indicated by either subjective account or observation made by others).

   3. Significant weight loss when not dieting or weight gain (e.g., a change of more than 5% of body weight in a month), or decrease or increase in appetite nearly every day.

   4. Insomnia or hypersomnia nearly every day.

   5. Psychomotor agitation or retardation nearly every day (observable by others, not merely subjective feelings of restlessness or being slowed down).

   6. Fatigue or loss of energy nearly every day.

   7. Feelings of worthlessness or excessive or inappropriate guilt (which may be delusional) nearly every day (not merely self-reproach or guilt about being sick).

   8. Diminished ability to think or concentrate, or indecisiveness, nearly every day (either by subjective account or as observed by others).

   9. Recurrent thoughts of death (not just fear of dying), recurrent suicidal ideation without a specific plan, or a suicide attempt or a specific plan for committing suicide.

B. The symptoms do not meet criteria for a Mixed Episode.

C. The symptoms cause clinically significant distress or impairment in social, occupational, or other important areas of functioning.

D. The symptoms are not due to the direct physiological effects of a substance (e.g., a drug of abuse, a medication) or a general medical condition (e.g., hypothyroidism).

E. The symptoms are not better accounted for by bereavement (ie, after the loss of a loved one); and the symptoms persist for longer than two months or are characterized by marked functional impairment, morbid preoccupation with worthlessness, suicidal ideation, psychotic symptoms, or psychomotor retardation.

---

*Major depressive disorder can be diagnosed upon the occurrence of a single major depressive episode. Recurrent major depressive disorder is diagnosed upon the occurrence of two or more major depressive episodes.

Source: American Psychiatric Association. *Diagnostic and Statistical Manual of Mental Disorders*. 4th ed. Washington, DC: American Psychiatric Press; 1994.[15]

It is clear that the severely depressed MS patient is likely to be fatigued, and treating the depression should improve fatigue. However, the reverse is not always true. The fact remains that, while there is overlap between severe fatigue in MS and depression, both symptoms can independently influence perceived health and quality of life.[20] Therefore, separate but overlapping treatment approaches for fatigue and depression should be implemented.

Anxiety and Fatigue

Anxiety in MS is common, with a reported frequency as high as 25% to 90%.[3] There have been few formal studies examining the relationship between anxiety and fatigue. One investigation of 101 MS patients did examine affective state and fatigue in association with neurologic impairment.[21] There did not appear to be a major effect of fatigue, in that controlling for the symptom of fatigue did not change the association among depression, anxiety, neurologic impairment, and quality of life. Nevertheless, it is reasonable to assume that the expenditure of energy and resources from unremitting anxiety in an individual with depleted reserves from MS will create added fatigue.

The Influence of Psychologic Factors on Fatigue

Regressional analyses in studies of large numbers of MS patients usually do not focus solely on the relationship between depressive symptoms and fatigue. Instead, there is a complex web of interactions between fatigue, depressive symptoms, other affective states, coping style (e.g., behavioral avoidance), and perceived mental and physical functioning, in addition to such physical factors as pain (Figure 1).[22] Exploring any one of these illness variables individually is unlikely to explain the role of fatigue in the disease state. In contrast, considering the group of factors as a whole, with different relative weighting, comes closer to capturing the nature of the complex fatigue experience in the individual with MS.

Among the psychosocial factors that contribute to fatigue and depression are feelings of control, helplessness, and illness perception.[23] Feelings of control lessen fatigue, whereas focusing on bodily sensations can exacerbate fatigue.[24] Individuals who feel they can create environments appropriate to their psychologic and physical needs have been shown to experience less fatigue and fatigue-related stress.[6] In those in medical groups who experience severe fatigue, fatigue correlates with low

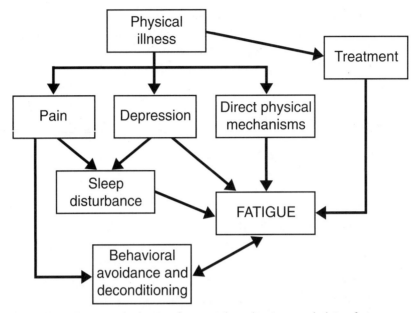

FIGURE 1   Integrated scheme of potential mechanisms underlying fatigue. Source: Wessely S, et al. *Chronic Fatigue and its Syndromes.* London, UK: Oxford University Press; 1999.[22]

positive affect, but does not correspond with elevated negative affect.[25,26] In a small study of 20 relapsing-remitting MS patients on interferon beta therapy who also had fatigue, there was a clear inverse relationship between fatigue severity and positive affect on the Positive and Negative Affect Scale, but no association between fatigue and negative affect.[27]

That the way patients perceive their illness is relevant to the fatigue experience was demonstrated in a study of 168 MS patients assessed using a range of measures of illness perception, self-esteem, anxiety, depression, and severity of MS.[28] Among many MS patients, the perception of their disease was much more central to the fatigue experience then either their ambulatory status or clinical disease subtype.

A sense of helplessness[14] is associated with the uncontrollable, unpredictable features of MS. This sense of helplessness is associated with depression and fatigue severity. It also correlates with higher EDSS scores, and may explain the relationship observed in some studies between fatigue and neurologic impairment.[14] In addition, a sense of hopelessness (e.g., a focus on the negative aspects of the future and thoughts of suicide) is associated with depression and a more progressive disease course.[29]

The close association between fatigue, personality traits,[30] psychologic factors, and chronic illness variables is not unique to MS. In other medical conditions, psychologic vulnerability has been shown to prolong illness recovery and, along with attributional and coping style, contribute to symptoms of persistent fatigue.[31–33] Given the complex nature of a disease that affects primarily young adults, can have a highly unpredictable course and cause a range of neurologic impairments, it is not surprising that there are many interactions between mood, chronic illness measures, and the symptom of fatigue.

Conclusions

Individuals with MS bring to their disease their own underlying personality and method of coping style. Thus, each person with MS-related fatigue has a unique set of physical and psychologic circumstances that contribute to this symptom. The fatigue that is caused by MS is further aggravated by depression, pain, and sleep disorders, and is also highly sensitive to the individual's coping pattern, attribution of illness style, and personality traits. The fact that these psychologic factors have powerful modulating effects on fatigue suggests that behavioral interventions may be helpful to selected MS fatigue patients.

References

1. Sadovnick AD, Remick RA, Allen J, et al. Depression and multiple sclerosis. *Neurology*. 1996;46:628-632.
2. Schubert DSP, Foliart RH. Increased depression in multiple sclerosis: a meta-analysis. *Psychosomatics*. 1993;34:124-130.
3. Minden S, Frumin M, Erb JL. Treatment of disorders of mood and affect in multiple sclerosis. In: Rudick RA, Cohen JA, eds. *Multiple Sclerosis Therapeutics*. 2nd ed. New York, NY: Martin Dunitz; 2003.
4. Chwastiak L, Ehde DM, Gibbons LE, Sullivan M, Bowen D, Kraft GH. Depressive symptoms and severity of illness in multiple sclerosis: epidemiologic study of a large community sample. *Am J Psychiatry*. 2002;159:1862-1868.
5. Friedberg F, Krupp LB. A comparison of cognitive behavioral treatment for chronic fatigue syndrome and primary depression. *Clin Infect Dis*. 1994;18(suppl 1):S105-S110.
6. Schwartz CE, Coulthard-Morris L, Zeng Q. Psychosocial correlates of fatigue in multiple sclerosis. *Arch Phys Med Rehabil*. 1996;77:165-170.
7. Ettinger AB, Weisbrot DM, Krupp LB, et al. Fatigue and depression in epilepsy. *J Epilepsy*. 1998;11:105-109.
8. Arnett PA, Higginson CI, Randlolf JJ. Depression in multiple sclerosis: relationship to planning ability. *J Int Neuropsychol Soc*. 2001;7:665-674.

9. Katon WY, Buchwald DS, Simon GE, Russo JE, Mease PJ. Psychiatric illness in patients with chronic fatigue and those with rheumatoid arthritis. *J Gen Intern Med.* 1991;6:277-285.

10. Voss WD, Arnett PA, Higginson CI, Randolph JJ, Campos MD, Dyck DG. Contributing factors to depressed mood in multiple sclerosis. *Arch Clin Neuropsychol.* 2002;17:103-115.

11. Bakshi R, Shaikh ZA, Miletich RS, et al. Fatigue in multiple sclerosis and its relationship to depression and neurologic disability. *Mult Scler.* 2000;6:181-185.

12. Egner A, Phillips VL, Vora R, Wiggers E. Depression, fatigue, and health-related quality of life among people with advanced multiple sclerosis: results from an exploratory telerehabilitation study. *Neurorehabilitation.* 2003;18:125-133.

13. Flachenecker P, Kumpfel T, Kallmann B, et al. Fatigue in multiple sclerosis: a comparison of different rating scales and correlation to clinical parameters. *Mult Scler.* 2002;8:523-526.

14. van der Werf SP, Evers A, Jongen PJ, Bleijenberg G. The role of helplessness as mediator between neurological disability, emotional instability, experienced fatigue and depression in patients with multiple sclerosis. *Mult Scler.* 2003;9:89-94.

15. American Psychiatric Association. *Diagnostic and Statistical Manual of Mental Disorders.* 4th ed. Washington, DC: American Psychiatric Press; 1994.

16. Mohr DC, Hart SL, Goldberg A. Effects of treatment for depression on fatigue in multiple sclerosis. *Psychosom Med.* 2003;65:542-547.

17. Whiting P, Bagnall AM, Sowden AJ, Cornell JE, Mulrow CD, Ramirez G. Interventions for the treatment and management of chronic fatigue syndrome: a systematic review. *JAMA.* 2001;286;1360-1368.

18. Schreurs KM, de Ridder DT, Bensing JM. Fatigue in multiple sclerosis: reciprocal relationships with physical disabilities and depression. *J Psychosom Res.* 2002;53:775-781.

19. Krupp LB, Coyle PK, Doscher C, et al. Fatigue therapy in multiple sclerosis: results of a double-blind, randomized, parallel trial of amantadine, pemoline, and placebo. *Neurology.* 1995;45:1956-61.

20. Amato MP, Ponziani G, Rossi F, Liedl CL, Stefanile C, Rossi L. Quality of life in multiple sclerosis: the impact of depression, fatigue and disability. *Mult Scler.* 2001;7:340-344.

21. Janssens AC, van Doorn PA, de Boer JB, et al. Anxiety and depression influence the relation between disability status and quality of life in multiple sclerosis. *Mult Scler.* 2003;9:397-403.

22. Wessely S, Hotopf M, Sharpe M. *Chronic Fatigue and its Syndromes.* London, UK: Oxford University Press; 1999.

23. Zonana-Nacach A, Roseman JM, McGwin G, et al. Systemic lupus erythematosus in three ethnic groups, VI: factors associated with fatigue within 5 years of criteria diagnosis. *Lupus.* 2000;9:101.

24. Vercoulen J, Hommes OR, Swanink C, et al. The measurement of fatigue in patients with multiple sclerosis: a multidimensional comparison with patients with chronic fatigue syndrome and healthy subjects. *Arch Neurol.* 1996,53:642-649.

25. Elkins LE, Pollina DA, Scheffer S, Krupp LB. Psychological states and neuropsychological performances in chronic Lyme disease. *Appl Neuropsych.* 1999;6:19-26.

26. Marshall PS, Watson D, Steinberg P, et al. An assessment of cognitive function and mood in chronic fatigue syndrome. *Biol Psych.* 1996;39:199-206.

27. Krupp LB, Christodoulou C, Madigan D, et al. The use of interferon beta-1a (IFN-beta-1a, Avonex) and modafinil to evaluate and treat cytokine-induced fatigue in multiple sclerosis. Presented at: the 127th Annual Meeting of the American Neurological Association; October 13-16, 2002; New York, NY.
28. Jopson NM, Moss-Morris R. The role of illness severity and illness representations in adjusting to multiple sclerosis. *J Psychosom Res.* 2003;54:503-511.
30. Merkelbach S, Konig J, Sittinger H. Personality traits in multiple sclerosis (MS) patients with and without fatigue experience. *Acta Neurol Scand.* 2003;107:195-201.
29. Patten SB, Metz LM. Hopelessness ratings in relapsing-remitting and secondary progressive multiple sclerosis. *Int J Psychiatry Med.* 2002;32:155-165.
31. Imboden JB, Canter A, Cluff LE. Convalescence from influenza: a study of the psychological and clinical determinants. *Arch Intern Med.* 1961;108:393-399.
32. Cohen S, Tyrrell AJ, Smith AP. Psychological stress and susceptibility to the common cold. *N Engl J Med.* 1991;325:606-612.
33. Cope H, David A, Pelosi A, Mann A. Predictors of chronic "postviral" fatigue. *Lancet.* 1994;344:864-868.

CHAPTER 6

Examination
and Diagnosis

A comprehensive workup for MS-related fatigue is essential to diagnosing fatigue and choosing an effective management strategy. The workup requires a detailed history from the patient and the family. In addition to a general and neurologic examination, laboratory testing to rule out other potential causes of fatigue is helpful. The evaluation should also include self-report measures of fatigue, sleep, pain, and depression/other mood disorders.

History

The history and physical examination should be designed to gain as full an understanding of the patient's physical and psychologic condition as possible, and to tease out any information that may indicate a cause of fatigue other than MS.

It is useful to distinguish between reports of pathologic fatigue (an overwhelming sense of tiredness or loss of energy that persists after rest) versus the transient, mild fatigue associated with otherwise healthy individuals. Fatigue should also be distinguished from excessive daytime sleepiness or affective disorders. The Epworth Sleepiness Scale (ESS) can help assess excessive daytime sleepiness (see Table 1).[1] In addition, it is often valuable to administer a brief inventory of mood, such as the Depression Subscale of the Multiple Sclerosis Quality of Life Inventory (MSQoL),[2] the Beck Depression Inventory (BDI),[3] or the Center for Epidemiologic Studies Depression Scale (CES-D).[4] One approach to administering these assessments is to ask patient to fill out the question-

TABLE 1   Epworth Sleepiness Scale (ESS)

The ESS can be used to detect symptoms of excessive daytime sleepiness (EDS), which may mimic fatigue. EDS may be a sign of a sleep disorder such as narcolepsy or sleep apnea syndrome. A score of ≥10 generally signifies the presence of moderate to severe EDS.

Indicate your chance of falling asleep under the following situations:

0 = no chance of dozing
1 = slight chance of dozing
2 = moderate chance of dozing
3 = high chance of dozing

Situation	Chance of Dozing
1. Sitting and reading	_____
2. Watching TV	_____
3. Sitting inactive in a public place (e.g., a theater or a meeting)	_____
4. As a passenger in a car for an hour without a break	_____
5. Lying down to rest in the afternoon when circumstances permit	_____
6. Sitting and talking to someone	_____
7. Sitting quietly after a lunch without alcohol	_____
8. In a car, while stopped for a few minutes in traffic	_____
TOTAL SCORE:	_____

Source: Johns MW. *Sleep.* 1991;14:540-545.[1]

naires while still in the waiting room. During the interview, specific questions about fatigue should include its onset (ie, whether it is acute or chronic), whether there are any variations during the day or night, the severity of the fatigue (which can be assessed using a self-report scale), and whether the fatigue is general or isolated to certain parts of the body (e.g., the upper or lower extremities).

The health care provider should also inquire whether the patient can identify any triggering factors that may worsen fatigue (e.g., heat, exercise, or personal or family stress) or situations and activities that can lessen fatigue (e.g., whether fatigue improves after exercise or rest). The guidelines for MS-related fatigue issued by the MS Council for Clinical Practice Guidelines include a fatigue diary that can be given to patients to help them identify potential triggers for fatigue and determine whether the timing or severity of fatigue varies (Table 2).[5] A copy of the diary or a similar tool can be given to patients when they initially complain of fatigue or tiredness, and reviewed during subsequent visits.

TABLE 2   MS Daily Activity Diary

Instructions

1. At the top of the day's diary, describe how you slept the night before.
2. Assign a number value from 1 to 10 (1 being very low and 10 being very high) for:
   - Your level of fatigue (**F**).
   - The value or importance of the activity you are doing (**V**).
   - The satisfaction you feel with your performance of the activity (**S**).

You can compute the "value" of an activity by comparing it to other activities you would like to do during the course of the day.

For example:

> **1 PM: F=7   V=3   S=2**
>
> **Activity:** Fixing lunch standing 15 minutes (hot)
>
> **Comment:** Blurred vision

3. Always describe the physical work done in the **Activity** section (e.g., stood to shower 10 minutes, went up 20 stairs, walked 200 feet).
4. Note the **external temperature** of the environment under **Activity**.
5. List under **Comments** all MS symptoms as they appear or worsen during the day, including cognitive problems, visual problems, weakness, dizziness, dragging foot, pain, numbness, burning, and so forth.
6. Make notes **every hour**.

Name: _____   Date: _____

Describe last night's sleep: _____

Time	F	V	S	Activity	Comment
6:00 AM					
7:00					
8:00					
9:00					
10:00					
11:00					
12:00 PM					
1:00					
2:00					
3:00					

(continued on next page)

TABLE 2   MS Daily Activity Diary (continued)

Time	F	V	S	Activity	Comment
4:00					
5:00					
6:00					
7:00					
8:00					
9:00					
10:00					
11:00					

Source: Multiple Sclerosis Council for Clinical Practice Guidelines. *Fatigue and Multiple Sclerosis: Evidence-Based Management Strategies for Fatigue in Multiple Sclerosis.* Washington, DC: Paralyzed Veterans of America; 1998.[5]

The history should include an assessment of professional activities and activities of daily living. The physician or nurse should inquire about the patient's occupation and level of stress at work, as well as any changes in occupational, educational, social, or personal activities.

While fatigue in an MS patient is most likely related to MS itself, other coexisting medical disorders could also produce fatigue and should be considered. Prominent diseases or conditions in which fatigue may be a symptom include malignancy,[6] chronic fatigue syndrome,[7] chronic kidney disease,[8] recent surgery,[9] Parkinson's disease,[10] chronic obstructive pulmonary disease,[11] human immunodeficiency virus infection,[12] or other acute or chronic infectious disorders such as hepatitis or influenza. The patient should also be asked about the presence of movement disorders such as restless legs syndrome or periodic limb movements of sleep. The patient's bed partner should be queried about the presence of any movement disorders during sleep, as well as the occurrence of sleep apneas/hypopneas.

In reviewing the medication history, it is necessary to consider the possible contribution to fatigue of medications such as benzodiazepines, muscle relaxants, antihistamines, and sedatives. (A list of medications that may cause or contribute to fatigue is given in Chapter 8.) The patient's immunomodulating therapies are also important factors, and should be assessed to determine whether an association can be established between interferon therapy and fatigue. Caffeine and alcohol intake should be determined, as excessive consumption may interfere with sleep patterns.

Questions on the patient's lifestyle should be designed to elicit information about relationships with family members, as stress and/or depression may be associated with fatigue. Careful attention should be paid to the patient's physical, emotional, and psychologic support network at home; if any of these are deemed to be insufficient, referral for appropriate care (e.g., occupational therapy, psychologic care, or a social work provider) should be given. The patient's degree of physical activity (exercise and recreational activities) should be assessed.

During the interview, the health care provider should observe the patient carefully for the presence of negative affect, apathy, or other signs that may be indicative of depression. Taking a psychologic history can be challenging. Patients may not be aware of depressive/fatigue symptoms, or they may have accepted them as a "normal" part of their lives. The physician should focus on the potential presence of depression or anxiety disorders; recent weight loss or gain, loss of appetite, feelings of sadness, or recent loss of interest in activities are all signs of depression.[13] The psychologic history should also ask about the patient's experience with alcohol or other drugs of abuse, prescription medication abuse, and a history of spousal abuse. If any of these are suspected, a psychiatric consultation is appropriate.

Physical Examination and Laboratory Testing

A comprehensive physical exam should be designed to rule out comorbid conditions that may be causing or contributing to fatigue. The exam should include a temperature/vital sign assessment, and a head, ear, eyes, nose, and throat evaluation to check for signs of lymph node enlargement, thyroid size, throat and ear redness or swelling, or otitis. Chest examination should check for the presence of abnormal heart and lung sounds that may indicate the need for cardiac/pulmonary testing. The skin should be examined carefully for evidence of rash or local erythema at injection sites, and the abdomen should be palpated and assessed for hepatosplenomegaly. A thorough neurologic examination should be conducted to assess for evidence of disease progression or abnormalities in affect.

A number of laboratory tests are available if a cause of fatigue other than MS is suspected. A nonexhaustive list of laboratory tests is shown in Table 3.[14] Routine laboratory tests should be used to exclude causes of fatigue such as infection and metabolic disease.[15] Imaging examinations such as conventional and functional magnetic resonance imaging (MRI) and positron emission tomography (PET) have been used to help diagnose MS and estimate disease progression. However, they are not indicated as part of the fatigue workup.

TABLE 3   Differential Diagnosis of Fatigue in the
MS Patient: Laboratory Testing

The following laboratory tests are useful if the physician has an index of suspicion for fatigue that is not related to MS:

Test	Assesses for:
Serial morning or afternoon temperatures	Infection, malignancy
Complete blood cell count and differential	Infection, malignancy
Sedimentation rate	Abscess, osteomyelitis, endocarditis, cancer, tuberculosis, mycosis, collagen-vascular disease
Electrolytes	Adrenal insufficiency, tuberculosis
Glucose	Diabetes mellitus
Blood urea nitrogen/creatinine	Renal failure
Calcium	Hyperparathyroidism, cancer, sarcoidosis
Total bilirubin	Hepatitis, hemolysis
Serum glutamic oxalocetic transaminase (SGOT)	Hepatocellular disease
Serum glutamic pyruvic transaminase (SGPT)	Hepatocellular abscess
Alkaline phosphatase	Obstructive liver disease
Creatine phosphokinase (CPK)	Muscle disease
Urinalysis	Renal disease, proteinuria
Posteroanterior lateral chest radiograph	Cardiopulmonary disease
Antinuclear antibodies	Systemic lupus erythematosus, other collagen-vascular disease
Thyroid stimulating hormone	Hypothyroidism
HIV antibody test	HIV/AIDS
Purified protein derivative	Tuberculosis
Hepatitis screen	Hepatitis
Lyme serologies	Lyme disease/postlyme syndrome

Source: Adapted from Morrison RE. *Obstet Gynecol Clin North Am.* 2001;28:225-235.[14]

Conclusions

The fatigue workup for the MS patient should be designed to determine specific triggers of fatigue and to systematically rule out other potential causes such as neurologic, cardiac, infectious, metabolic, and neoplastic disease. Careful attention should be paid to the patient's psychologic history to identify or rule out affective disorders such as depression. Because of the high prevalence of fatigue in the MS patient, it should be considered a diagnosis of inclusion; a careful patient history and appropriate laboratory testing can be used to rule out other suspected causes.

References

1. Johns MW. A new method for measuring daytime sleepiness: the Epworth Sleepiness Scale. *Sleep*. 1991;14:540-545.
2. National Multiple Sclerosis Society. *Multiple Sclerosis Quality of Life Inventory: A User's Manual*. New York, NY: National Multiple Sclerosis Society; 1997.
3. Beck AT, Ward CH, Mendelson M, Mock J, Erbaugh J. An inventory for measuring depression. *Arch Gen Psychiatry*. 1961;4:561-571.
4. Radloff LS. The CES-D scale: A self-report depression scale for research in the general population. *Applied Psychological Measurement*. 1997;1:385-401.
5. Multiple Sclerosis Council for Clinical Practice Guidelines. *Fatigue and Multiple Sclerosis: Evidence-Based Management Strategies for Fatigue in Multiple Sclerosis*. Washington, DC: Paralyzed Veterans of America; 1998.
6. Curt GA, Breitbart W, Cella D, et al. Impact of cancer-related fatigue on the lives of patients: new findings from the Fatigue Coalition. *Oncologist*. 2000;5:353-360.
7. Schluederberg A, Straus SE, Peterson P, et al. NIH conference: chronic fatigue syndrome research: definition and medical outcome assessment. *Ann Intern Med*. 1992;117:325-331.
8. NKF/DOQI. Clinical practice guidelines for the treatment of anemia of chronic renal failure: National Kidney Foundation Dialysis Outcomes Quality Initiative: 2000 update. *Am J Kidney Dis*. 2001;37(suppl 1):S186-S206.
9. DeCherney AH, Bachmann G, Isaacson K, Gall S. Postoperative fatigue negatively impacts the daily lives of patients recovering from hysterectomy. *Obstet Gynecol*. 2002;99:51-57.
10. Friedman JH, Friedman H. Fatigue in Parkinson's disease: a nine-year follow-up. *Mov Disord*. 2001;16:1120-1122.
11. Woo K. A pilot study to examine the relationships of dyspnoea, physical activity and fatigue in patients with chronic obstructive pulmonary disease. *J Clin Nurs*. 2000;9:526-533.
12. Adinolfi A. Assessment and treatment of HIV-related fatigue. *J Assoc Nurses AIDS Care*. 2001;12(suppl):29-34.
13. American Psychiatric Association. *Diagnostic and Statistical Manual of Mental Disorders*. 4th ed. Washington, DC: American Psychiatric Press; 1994.
14. Morrison RE, Keating HJ. Fatigue in primary care. *Obstet Gynecol Clin North Am*. 2001;28:225-237.
15. Krupp LB. Fatigue in MS: pathophysiology, measurement and management. *CNS Drugs*. 2003;17:225-234.

CHAPTER 7

Nonpharmacologic Approaches

Multiple sclerosis-related fatigue requires a comprehensive management strategy that should incorporate a range of nonpharmacologic interventions. Patients can be greatly helped by an exercise plan, nutritional counseling, energy-conservation strategies, and cooling strategies for heat-induced fatigue (whether or not it is related to exercise). This chapter discusses the basic principles of nonpharmacologic management of fatigue. The recommendations discussed here vary in the degree to which they have been explored specifically for MS-related fatigue; therefore, there is a greater level of evidence for some strategies than for others. Unfortunately not all of the recommended interventions have been tested in randomized, controlled trials. Nevertheless, all of these strategies incorporate common-sense approaches to overall physical and mental well-being that can be expected to reduce the deleterious effects of fatigue. The few available controlled studies that have been conducted have tended to support these nonpharmacologic approaches to management.

Exercise

Exercise provides numerous benefits to individuals with MS, including decreases in risk factors for cardiovascular disease, reduction in obesity, and improvement in mood.[1] On the contrary, limiting physical activity contributes to muscle weakness and worsening aerobic capacity, which can cause fatigue, worsen existing fatigue, and make it more difficult to reverse fatigue symptoms.

No innate symptoms or qualities of MS specifically contraindicate exercise. It has been demonstrated that MS patients exhibit a normal cardiovascular response to exercise, and that they can exercise sufficiently to improve their fitness levels.[2,3] Exercise has proven beneficial in other chronic disease states such as cancer,[4] and similar effects can be expected for people with MS.[5]

Several recent studies have examined the effects of exercise on fatigue, as well as closely related measures such as vitality and overall cardiovascular health. These trials used various study designs, making it difficult to draw comparisons among trials. However, all have demonstrated at least some degree of improvement with regard to fatigue and/or vitality. One short-term trial randomized 26 patients with moderate disability (EDSS mean, 4.5-4.6) to an exercise training program or to no exercise intervention as part of an inpatient rehabilitation program.[5] All patients were able to pedal on a free-standing bicycle ergometer and had no history of cardiovascular, respiratory, or other conditions that precluded participation in the training program. A graded maximal exercise test, tests of lung function, and various questionnaires that included the Fatigue Severity Scale (FSS) and Medical Outcomes Survey Short Form 36 (SF-36) were administered at baseline and at the end of 4 weeks. Also included were 26 healthy, mostly sedentary persons who served as controls. Baseline testing showed that the levels of fatigue on the FSS were 60 to 67% higher in the MS groups compared with the healthy, but sedentary controls.

Those assigned to the exercise program participated in five supervised training sessions per week over 3 to 4 weeks, with each session consisting of 30 minutes of bicycle exercise training. The patients assigned to exercise training showed significant increases on respiratory measures of forced vital capacity and peak expiratory flow rate. A 17% increase in sport-related activity was also demonstrated. Of the scales used to measure fatigue, there was a trend toward reduced fatigue on the FSS in the exercise group compared with the no-exercise group (–14% versus –4%; $P=0.09$); however, there was a significant increase in the vitality subscale of the SF-36 in the exercise group, as well as a significant increase in social functioning. No significant increase was seen on either of these scales in the no-exercise group.

The results showed that a short-term exercise program can be sufficient to impact fatigue and vitality scores in MS patients with a high baseline level of fatigue, by counteracting the effects of detraining secondary to fatigue. The lack of a significant effect on the FSS was deemed potentially related to the short duration of the study, which may not have been long enough to exhibit significantly marked changes. Alternatively, the FSS may not have been sensitive enough to detect changes in fatigue over a short period of time.[5] A longer, 15-week graded exercise program showed significant reductions in the fatigue category of the Profile of Mood States (POMS) at week 10, but again, no significant reduction on the FSS.[3] In this study also, it was suggested that the FSS may be insufficiently sensitive to changes over time.

The effects on fatigue of a longer-term outpatient rehabilitation program were examined in a trial of 46 patients with chronic progressive MS.[6] In this study, 20 patients were randomized to rehabilitation services for 5 hours, 1 day per week, over the course of 1 year. They were compared with 26 patients in a nontreatment group who were assigned to a waiting list for rehabilitation. The program integrated physical therapy with supportive services to maintain physical function, as well as occupational therapy and nutrition services. Fatigue, measured as an item on the 26-item MS-Related Symptom Checklist, was significantly reduced in the treatment group compared with the waiting group ($P=0.004$).[6]

Practical Considerations for Exercise

Unfortunately, few resources offer specific exercise guidelines for the MS patient, to alleviate fatigue and improve well-being.[1] Thus, physicians must use careful clinical judgment in assessing the patient and assigning an exercise program. Programs should be tailored to meet individual circumstances, taking into account medications, exacerbations, and recovery stages.[1] For the severely disabled patient, exercises to maximize independence, including strengthening muscles used for activities of daily living and exercises for balance, coordination, and range of motion, may be most appropriate.[7]

Health care providers must assess how new the patient is to exercise and give an appropriate evaluation of cardiovascular and overall health risk, as well as any non-MS-related conditions that may pose additional health risks, such as asthma. Any exercise program must be designed with the patient's level of physical activity in mind, and adjustments must be made that take into account the patient's level of disability (e.g., use of special shoes, use of foot straps for stationary cycles). Thorough neurologic and musculoskeletal examinations should be performed that take into account factors such as gait, balance, and degree of spasticity. A physical therapist should be consulted initially and used periodically to monitor the patient's progress. A hierarchical program that is designed to meet the individual needs of the patient should then be developed, with patients progressing at their own pace through the different stages (passive range of motion, active resistance, specific strengthening, integrated strength exercises, and increases in the amount of time devoted to cardiovascular workouts).[8]

People tend to have a low degree of adherence to exercise programs, whether or not they have MS. Therefore, when initially discussing an exercise program, the physician must make every effort to "sell" the program to the patient, conveying its importance and giving the same weight to exercise as to any pharmacologic therapy. The exercise program should be presented as a structured regimen that includes details such as the number of days each exercise should be performed, the amount of time spent on each exercise, and the specific number of repetitions performed. In the author's experience, providing a prescription for the exercise program gives additional authority to the program and underscores its importance.

Patients also should receive positive reinforcement for completing an exercise program. Asking the spouse or partner to provide a special reward (dinner out, etc.) at the end of a month of exercise is an important way of sustaining morale and encouraging the activity. Offering acknowledgment or adapting cognitive-behavioral methods can aid in increasing patient adherence to an exercise program. Table 1 summarizes some adherence techniques that can be discussed with the patient.

Cooling Programs

Given the association between heat, fatigue, and deficits in nerve impulse conduction, heat sensitivity is a major factor to take into account for MS patients regardless of whether they are assigned to an exercise program.[9] Several small studies have shown that the use of cooling garments can effectively decrease fatigue in MS patients. In a series of case studies designed to assess the perceived impact of fatigue with the use of a cooling suit, eight individuals reported a reduction in fatigue on the Fatigue Impact Scale (FIS), as well as reduced sense of fatigue or affective problems related to fatigue on patient diaries and interviews.[10]

In a crossover study that randomized patients to active cooling (7° C) or sham cooling (26° C) for 60-minute periods with a head-vest cooling garment, active cooling was associated with improvements in fatigue on the Shortened Fatigue Questionnaire, an instrument that rates four fatigue-related questions on a 7-point scale.[11] The improvement in fatigue was associated with decreases in nitric oxide (NO) production, which

TABLE 1	Ensuring Patient Adherence to an Exercise Program

The following will help the fatigue patient adhere to an exercise program over the long term:

- *Make sure the patient has the right equipment:* Depending on their level of mobility, patients may need adaptive equipment such as special footwear, walkers, or safety guards that can be attached to exercise equipment. The physician should consult with a physical therapist to assess the patient's needs in this regard.

- *Use a pyramid approach:* The exercise plan should be based on a pyramid approach, both for muscle fitness and aerobic fitness. With a pyramid approach to muscle fitness, the patient should start with simple range-of-motion exercises, gradually working up to strength-training exercises that involve all major muscle groups. For aerobic fitness, the patient can start by slowly increasing the number of normal daily activities, moving on to mild recreational activities, and eventually to a structured exercise program. An exercise program can involve activities such as walking, treadmill work, or cycling for 30 to 45 minutes three to four times per week.

- *Have the patient choose enjoyable activities:* Allowing patients to choose activities that they enjoy will give them a better chance of succeeding over the long-term.

- *Work with the patient on exercise planning:* Encourage the patient to get enough sleep the night before, and to plan exercise activities during times when fatigue is less severe. A fatigue diary (see Chapter 6) can be useful in identifying such times. Instruct the patient never to exercise to the point of exhaustion.

- *Make exercise a "prescription":* Treat your discussions on exercise with the patient with the same degree of gravity that you would pharmaceutical prescriptions.

- *Encourage patients to reward themselves:* Encourage patients to set exercise goals and give themselves small rewards for achieving these goals.

leads to improvement in nerve conduction; active cooling was associated with a 41% decrease in mean leukocyte NO production ($P=0.004$).

For the patient engaging in exercise, a water program can be considered to prevent overheating. A water temperature of less than 85° F has been recommended[12]; however, there is evidence from one case study that higher temperatures (94° F) may not induce fatigue.[13] In addition to its cooling effects, the buoyancy and viscosity of water can facilitate movement, alleviate problems with balance, and provide resistance for muscle strengthening.[13]

If a water exercise program is neither desirable for the patient nor easily accessible, other options include precooling prior to exercise and the use of cooling garments during exercise. In a study of six MS patients with demonstrated thermosensitivity in which each subject performed an exercise test with or without precooling, the subjects performed better and had lower levels of fatigue following the precooled trial.[14] Precooling consisted of immersion to the level of the suprailiac crest for 30 minutes in a water bath of 16–17° C. Fatigue was assessed via FIS scores, which were significantly lower in the precooled group than in the noncooled group immediately following exercise (FIS mean, 23 versus 30; $P<0.05$).[14]

Nutrition

No special diet specifically treats fatigue. However, developing a solid nutrition program can help maintain overall health, increase energy reserves, improve sleep, and reduce tiredness.

MS patients who are fatigued can be offered nutritional counseling to evaluate their dietary habits and to educate them on the cornerstones of healthy nutrition. For patients who are overweight, their excess weight can contribute to fatigue and deconditioning. Patients may also be underweight, due to the state of "high metabolic demand" that results from battling a chronic illness such as MS. The following are some nutritional guidelines that can be discussed with patients:

- *Avoid refined sugars and other sweets:* Excess sugar can alter blood glucose levels, increasing tiredness as glucose levels "spike" and then drop.
- *Ensure adequate hydration:* Dehydration can increase feelings of fatigue. Drinking adequate fluids (preferably water) should be encouraged. This is especially important following exercise, as dehydration may not always be apparent. Potential bladder problems should be taken into account in making recommendations for fluid intake; drinking too much liquid can create a need for nighttime bathroom trips, thus interfering with sleep, which can be another potential contributor to daytime fatigue. A prescription for oxybutynin (Ditropan-XL®) or another agent to control overactive bladder should be considered in these cases.
- *Limit consumption of caffeine and avoid tobacco:* Both caffeine and tobacco act as central nervous system (CNS) stimulants, and can interfere with sleep. Both should be assessed during the patient interview. If a smoking-cessation plan is needed, the selective norepinephrine reuptake inhibitor bupropion (available as Zyban® for smoking cessation and Wellbutrin-XL™ for depression) can be considered, as it

has the added benefit of antidepressant activity, and at least one report has supported its benefits for improving fatigue.[15]

- *Ensure quality nutrition:* A balanced diet should include foods that are high in vitamins, minerals, protein, and complex carbohydrates. High-quality protein (fish, poultry, and lean meat) can help the patient preserve muscle mass, while complex carbohydrates (such as potatoes, whole-grain foods, and legumes) can help stabilize blood sugar and energy levels. A diet with adequate fiber can help avoid constipation, which also may contribute to feelings of fatigue.

  In premenopausal women and those for whom there is a likelihood of blood loss (e.g., postsurgical patients), supplemental iron may be considered, as there is a clear association between fatigue and anemic states.[16] Several commercial iron supplements are available, generally containing about 200 mg/d of elemental iron.[16]

- *Eat smaller meals:* Eating smaller meals throughout the day instead of three large meals can also help stabilize the patient's energy levels, and avoid feelings of fatigue and lethargy.

- *Limit alcohol intake:* Although alcohol is not specifically proscribed for the fatigue patient, it acts as a CNS depressant and can interfere with sleep, increasing feelings of daytime tiredness and fatigue. In addition, alcohol interacts with a number of medications that the patient may be taking for other MS symptoms (e.g., benzodiazepines).

- *Exercise regularly:* Regular exercise can help stimulate the appetite. It also helps maintain a healthy weight.

- *Assess the patient's use of "herbal" or "alternative" therapies:* Manufacturers of supplements and herbal products often make claims that these products can fight fatigue. With the exception of iron supplements, which can treat fatigue related to anemia, there is no evidence that these alternative therapies are useful for fatigue. The use of such products should be discouraged.

Principles of Energy Conservation

Principles of energy conservation, or "energy-effectiveness strategies," have not been subjected to extensive evaluation as part of a strategy for MS fatigue management. Nonetheless, the few studies available are supportive of an energy conservation approach. One such study evaluated the effect of a six-session, 2-hour per week energy course taught by occupational therapists to 54 patients with MS-related fatigue. Reductions in fatigue were seen on the FIS, combined with improvements in quality of life and assessments of self-efficacy on the Self-Efficacy Gauge, a measure of the patient's confidence in the ability to perform specific behaviors.[17]

Energy conservation was also effective in reducing fatigue as measured by the FIS in an 8-week energy conservation program involving 37 patients with progressive MS. Patients were randomized either to an experimental energy conservation program or an 8-week period of traditional treatment, using a crossover design study. The total FIS and the FIS subscale scores (physical, cognitive, and psychosocial) significantly declined during the experimental treatment program but not during the control period. Improvement was also maintained 8 weeks later in those subjects available for repeat evaluation.[18]

These data support the use of occupational therapy referrals in helping patients learn energy conservation techniques as a means of reducing fatigue. Some specific recommendations regarding energy conservation are given in the Appendix.[19]

Conclusions

Nonpharmacologic interventions are an essential component of therapy for the fatigued MS patient, as they can have significant benefits in reducing or eliminating both secondary and primary MS fatigue. Unfortunately, the interventions that are necessary, including exercise, changes in diet and nutrition, and adoption of energy-effective strategies, all require long-term commitments and lifestyle changes that make them difficult to integrate into patient routines. Therefore, it is up to the physician and the entire health care team to be especially vigilant in making sure that the patient adheres to nonpharmacologic therapy recommendations.

References

1. Sutherland G, Andersen MB. Exercise and multiple sclerosis: physiological, psychological, and quality of life issues. *J Sports Med Phys Fitness.* 2001;41:421-432.
2. Stuifbergen AK. Physical activity and perceived health status in persons with multiple sclerosis. *J Neurosci Nurs.* 1997;29:238-243.
3. Petajan JH, Gappmaier E, White AT, et al. Impact of aerobic training on fitness and quality of life in multiple sclerosis. *Ann Neurol.* 1996;39:432-441.
4. Dimeo FC. Effects of exercise on cancer-related fatigue. *Cancer.* 2001;92:1689-1693.
5. Mostert S, Kesselring J. Effects of a short-term exercise training program on aerobic fitness, fatigue, health perceptions, and activity level of subjects with multiple sclerosis. *Mult Scler.* 2002;8:161-168.
6. DiFabio RP, Soderberg J, Choi T, Hansen CR, Schapiro RT. Extended outpatient rehabilitation: its influence on symptom frequency, fatigue, and func-

tional status for persons with progressive multiple sclerosis. *Arch Phys Med Rehabil.* 1998;79:141-146.

7. DiFabio RP, Choi T, Soderberg J, Hansen CR. Health-related quality of life for patients with progressive multiple sclerosis: influence of rehabilitation. *Phys Ther.* 1997;77:1704-1716.

8. Petajan JH, White AT. Recommendations for physical activity in patients with multiple sclerosis. *Sports Medicine.* 1999;27:179-191.

9. Guthrie TC, Nelson DA. Influence of temperature changes on multiple sclerosis: critical review of mechanisms and research potential. *J Neurol Sci.* 1995;129:1-8.

10. Flesner G, Lindencrona C. The cooling suit: case studies of its influence on fatigue among eight individuals with multiple sclerosis. *J Adv Nurs.* 2002;37:541-550.

11. Beenakker EAC, Oparina TI, Hartgring A, Teelken A, Arutjunyan AV, De Keyser J. Cooling garment treatment in MS: clinical improvement and decrease in leukocyte NO production. *Neurology.* 2001;57:892-894.

12. Woods DA. Aquatic exercise programs for patients with multiple sclerosis. *Clin Kinesiology.* 1992;46(3):14-20.

13. Peterson C. Exercise in 94° F water for a patient with multiple sclerosis. *Phys Ther.* 2001;81:1049-1058.

14. White AT, Wilson TE, Davis SL, Petajan JH. Effect of precooling on physical performance in multiple sclerosis. *Mult Scler.* 2000;6:176-180.

15. Duffy JC, Campbell J. Bupropion for the treatment of fatigue associated with multiple sclerosis. *Psychosomatics.* 1994;35:170-171.

16. NKF/DOQI. Clinical practice guidelines for the treatment of anemia of chronic renal failure: National Kidney Foundation Dialysis Outcomes Quality Initiative: 2000 update. *Am J Kidney Dis.* 2001;37(suppl 1):S186-S206.

17. Mathiowetz V, Matuska KM, Murphy ME. Efficacy of an energy conservation course for persons with multiple sclerosis. *Arch Phys Med Rehabil.* 2001;82:449-456.

18. Vanage SM, Gilbertson KK, Mathiowetz V. Effects of an energy conservation course on fatigue impact for persons with progressive multiple sclerosis. *Am J Occup Ther.* 2003;57:315-323.

19. Schapiro RT. *Symptom Management in Multiple Sclerosis.* 4th ed. New York, NY: Demos Medical Publishing Co.; 2003.

CHAPTER 8
Pharmacologic Management

Nonpharmacologic measures should be considered first-line therapies for fatigue. These include exercise, proper nutrition, and energy conservation strategies. Nevertheless, if the patient does not respond or responds inadequately to these measures, adding pharmacologic therapy is often a necessary next step. In patients with overwhelming and severe fatigue who are unlikely to engage in exercise, medication should be considered a first-line option. This chapter discusses drug therapy options for MS-related fatigue, including issues related to medication management for the control of other symptoms and those surrounding immunomodulator use.

Adjustment of Symptomatic Medications

A 55-year-old nurse with secondary progressive MS was experiencing severe fatigue, spasticity, and painful leg spasms at night, which disrupted her sleep. She required assistance with transfers, and was either confined to a wheelchair or to her bed most of the day. High doses of baclofen (in the range of 180 mg/day) were necessary to control the painful spasms. However, her fatigue, which had been severe at baseline, became overwhelming with the increases in oral baclofen, and was further complicated by lethargy and mental slowing. The patient underwent baclofen pump insertion and was able to discontinue oral baclofen. At an intrathecal dose of 100 mcg/day, she was able to sleep pain free without spasms at night. During the day, her muscle tone was significantly reduced, yet she was mentally alert, no longer lethargic, and her fatigue was much improved.

The preceding case illustrates the fatiguing effects that can result from medications used to control other symptoms of MS. Multiple sclerosis patients often require medications that control spasticity, tremor, bowel or bladder dysfunction, and pain. They may also be taking medications for other diseases/conditions that may be related to or independent of MS, including depression and anxiety.

Table 1[1] is a partial list of medications that can have sedating properties that contribute to fatigue. Medications that carry a high risk of sedation and/or muscle weakness and that can cause or exacerbate fatigue include those used for analgesia (hydrocodone and other opioids); muscle relaxants (carisoprodal, diazepam and other benzodiazepines, tizanidine, and baclofen); and sedative/hypnotic medications (benzodiazepines and benzodiazepine receptor agonists such as zolpidem). As part of the fatigue workup, the health care provider needs to be aware of all medications that the patient is taking, noting the changes in regimens (as well as the reason for the regimen change) in the patient's chart. It is important to determine not simply what was prescribed at the prior visit, but to determine, using the individual's family as a resource if necessary, what the individual with MS is truly taking (including any over-the-counter medications and/or "alternative" therapies). Patients should also be asked to keep track of medications, and to pay careful attention to any perceived association between medication use and feelings of fatigue.

In general, initiation of medication should begin by starting at the lowest possible dose and titrating up slowly so that the patient can adjust to medications that may be sedating. Dosing of sedating medications in the evening can reduce daytime fatigue and help facilitate sleep.

Issues With Immunomodulator Therapy

Fatigue in association with other flu-like symptoms (e.g., fever and chills) can develop with interferon beta therapy (see Chapter 4). These symptoms usually abate after several months, but in some individuals, persist for longer periods. Flu-like symptoms, including fatigue, can develop the day after either subcutaneous or intramuscular injection, and may persist for 1 or more days. The reaction can be treated with a combination of acetaminophen and ibuprofen for pain and fever control. It is useful to take both medications prior to the interferon beta injection, several hours after the injection, and the morning following the injection.

In addition to acetaminophen or ibuprofen, the wake-promoting agent modafinil can reduce cytokine-induced fatigue. In a small study

TABLE 1 Pharmacologic Agents That May Cause/Contribute to Fatigue in the MS Patient

Drug	Used for:	Examples
Analgesics	Pain control	Butalbital, hydrocodone (Vicodin®), oxycodone (Oxycontin®)
Interferon therapies	Reducing MS exacerbations	Interferon beta-1a (Avonex®, Rebif®); interferon beta-1b (Betaseron®)
Muscle relaxants	Spasticity, muscle strain, anxiety disorders	Tizanidine (Zanaflex®), baclofen (oral or through an intrathecal pump); carisoprodal (Soma®)
Sedatives/ hypnotics	Sleep aids, anxiety, muscle relaxation	Alprazolam (Xanax®), clonazepam (Klonopin®); diazepam (Valium®); zolpidem (Ambien®)
Anticonvulsants	Seizure control; pain control; depression or anxiety	Carbamazepine (Tegretol®); divalproex (Depakote®); gabapentin (Neurontin®)
Antidepressants	Depression and anxiety disorders	Clomipramine (Anafranil®); nefazodone (Serzone®); sertraline (Zoloft®)
Antihistamines	Allergies, hay fever	Diphenhydramine (Benadryl® or other over-the-counter allergy medicines); cetirizine (Zyrtec®)
Antipsychotics	Schizophrenia, psychoses	Clozapine (Clozaril®); risperidone (Risperdal®)
Hormone therapies	Hormone replacement, contraception	Medroxyprogesterone (Depo-Provera®)

Source: Multiple Sclerosis Council for Clinical Practice Guidelines. *Fatigue and Multiple Sclerosis: Evidence-Based Management Strategies for Fatigue in Multiple Sclerosis.* Washington, DC: Paralyzed Veterans of America; 1998.[1]

involving 18 patients, eight of whom reported increased fatigue following weekly intramuscular injections of interferon beta-1a, the use of modafinil significantly reduced fatigue scores on the Fatigue Severity Scale (FSS) ($P<0.05$), and improved positive affect scores on the Positive and Negative Affect Scale (PANAS).[2] In this study, modafinil was given at a starting dose of 100 mg 48 hours after the interferon beta-1a injection, and titrated to 200 mg daily after 3 days. Low doses of prednisone also can be used to control persistent flu-like symptoms following inteferon beta therapy.[3]

Glatiramer acetate has a lower incidence of malaise, fatigue, and other flu-like effects compared with the interferon betas. In the controlled, premarketing clinical trials of this agent, a flu-like syndrome was reported by 19% of patients.[4] Thus, in patients who are naïve to immunomodulator therapy, if severe fatigue is a major concern, the fact that glatiramer acetate has a reduced association with fatigue may be a factor to consider when the patient and physician choose a therapy.

Medications Used to Treat MS-Related Fatigue

Pharmacologic therapy is critical in the treatment of MS-related fatigue. While no medication has been specifically approved by the US Food and Drug Administration (FDA) to treat MS-related fatigue, several agents have been used over the past 2 decades, demonstrating varying degrees of benefit (Table 2). Of these, the greatest degree of chemical information is available on the antiviral agent amantadine, the central nervous system

TABLE 2   Drugs Commonly Used to Treat MS-Related Fatigue (Adult Doses)

Drug	Starting Dose	Usual Maintenance Dose	Usual Maximum Dose	Side Effects
Amantadine (Symmetrel®)	100 mg per day in the morning	100 mg twice per day	300 mg per day	Insomnia, vivid dreams
Modafinil (Provigil®)	100 mg per day in the morning	200 mg per day in the morning, or 100 mg in the morning and 100 mg at lunchtime	200 mg per day (some people might respond well to higher doses)	Headache, insomnia
Pemoline (Cylert®)	18.75 mg per day in the morning	18.75–56.25 mg per day	93.75 mg per day	Irritability, restlessness, insomnia, potential liver problems
Bupropion, sustained release (Wellbutrin-XL™)	150 mg per day in the morning	150 mg per day	450 mg per day	Agitation, anxiety, insomnia
Fluoxetine (Prozac®)	20 mg per day in the morning	20–80 mg per day	80 mg per day	Weakness, nausea, insomnia
Venlafaxine (Effexor-XR®)	75 mg per day in the morning	75–225 mg per day	225 mg per day	Weakness, nausea, dizziness

(CNS) stimulant pemoline, and the wake-promoting agent modafinil.[5-10] Other agents that have been examined include the aminopyridines, antidepressants, and transdermal histamine/caffeine.

Amantadine

Amantadine is approved by the FDA for the prevention and treatment of influenza type A infection and for the management of parkinsonian and drug-related extrapyramidal reactions.[11] Its antiparkinsonian activity is related to its ability to block presynaptic dopamine reuptake and to directly stimulate postsynaptic receptors.[11] Its effect on MS-related fatigue is possibly related to these dopaminergic mechanisms.

Amantadine has been evaluated for the treatment of MS-related fatigue in at least four controlled trials, all of which administered the agent in a dose of 100 mg twice a day to the active-therapy groups.[5-8] Three of these were randomized, controlled trials conducted in the 1980s that compared amantadine with placebo,[5-7] with each trial using a different evaluation scale to assess the effects on fatigue symptoms.

The first trial, published in 1985,[5] was undertaken following the observation that an MS patient taking amantadine for influenza showed improvement in MS-related symptoms. Following an open-label investigation of amantadine, in which 14 of 18 treated patients achieved a positive response, the investigators enrolled 32 patients in a double-blind, crossover comparison of amantadine and placebo. A 4-point fatigue scale (marked, moderate, mild, or no improvement) was used to evaluate response to treatment after 3 months of therapy. Amantadine treatment improved fatigue, as evidenced by a significant difference in the number of patients reporting any degree of improvement (62.5% versus 21.8% for placebo; $P=0.0005$). At the end of the trial, no patient expressed a preference for placebo over amantadine.

In a second study, amantadine was compared with placebo in 29 MS patients who had symptomatic fatigue for at least 3 months prior to study entry.[6] This randomized, crossover trial consisted of two 4-week treatment periods, with a 2-week washout between treatments. Fatigue was measured by patient self-rating on seven indices, each with a 5-point scale ranging from 1 (poor) to 5 (excellent). Amantadine treatment did not significantly improve the overall fatigue score compared with placebo (3.18 versus 2.96; $P=0.058$). However, in a separate analysis of each of the indices used in the study, significant differences were seen in general energy level, concentration and memory, well-being, and the ability to solve problems. No significant improvement was seen in muscle strength, motivation level, or the ability to finish a task. Eight of the 22 patients who completed the study reported that they felt less fatigued while taking amantadine.

The largest of these three studies was a 10-week, multicenter Canadian trial that included 115 patients with a 3-month history of "chronic persistent fatigue."[7] A 50-mm Visual Analog Scale for Fatigue (VAS-F) was used to assess daily fatigue. Activities (selected by each patient) most affected by fatigue and 13 activities of daily living were also evaluated weekly by a VAS. The study consisted of a 2-week placebo run-in period, with two 3-week treatment periods separated by a 2-week washout.

A crossover analysis of variance detected a significant period effect, with fatigue significantly greater in the 2-week baseline period (31.6 mm) compared with the 2-week washout period (27 mm). This effect was seen regardless of the treatment (placebo or amantadine) during the first period. To accommodate this period effect, an analysis of covariance model was fitted for each of the 3 treatment weeks using the mean of the two baseline fatigue scores as a covariant.

Amantadine decreased fatigue in this study; however, the improvement was only statistically significant at week 1 ($P<0.01$). Amantadine use resulted in a significant mean decrease in the effect of fatigue on selected activities compared with placebo at each of the 3 weeks ($P<0.05$), and when the overall treatment effect was analyzed ($P<0.01$). The percentage of patients reporting adverse effects was 57% with amantadine and 54% with placebo. Of adverse effects specifically monitored in the study, only insomnia was reported significantly more often with amantadine (13 patients) than with placebo (four patients; $P=0.029$).

Another study evaluated the pharmacologic treatment of fatigue in 119 patients with clinically definite MS, using the FSS and MS-Specific Fatigue Scale (MS-FS) as the outcome measures. This was a multicenter, parallel-group trial in which patients were randomized to either amantadine (n=39), pemoline (n=37), or placebo (n=43) treatment arms.[8] Patients had clinically significant fatigue (scores of ≥4 on the FSS) and were ambulatory. Exclusion criteria included the recent use of fatigue-promoting medications and severe depression. Treatment effect was assessed before, during, and at the end of treatment using the FSS and MS-FS. Patients were also asked to give verbal self-reports at the end of 8 weeks of treatment and 2 weeks after treatment ended.

Amantadine significantly decreased fatigue on the MS-FS compared with placebo ($P=0.037$). In addition, following the 2-week washout period at the end of the study, 79% of amantadine patients versus 52% of placebo patients stated that they felt better on study medication compared with no treatment ($P=0.03$). The FSS scores were not significantly different for amantadine compared with placebo, although there was a significant difference compared with baseline.

Pemoline

Pemoline, which is indicated for the treatment of attention deficit hyperactivity disorder, is a CNS stimulant unrelated to other stimulants such as methylphenidate.[12] Its effects usually peak about 4 hours postdose, and last up to 8 hours.

Two randomized, controlled clinical trials have evaluated the use of pemoline for MS-related fatigue. In the study discussed above that compared amantadine, pemoline, and placebo, pemoline was started at a dose of 18.75 mg/day at week 1 and titrated to 56.25 mg/day by week 3.[8] No significant difference between pemoline and placebo was seen on the MS-FS or FSS in this study. In addition, significantly more patients in this study showed a preference for amantadine than for pemoline (79% versus 32%; $P=0.035$). More patients also expressed a preference for placebo than for pemoline (52% versus 32%), although this difference did not reach statistical significance.

More favorable results with pemoline were observed in another study that used somewhat higher doses. Pemoline was compared with placebo in a two-center, crossover trial of 46 patients with severe fatigue at a dose of 75 mg/day in a 4-week dose-escalation study that used a 50-mm VAS as the assessment tool.[9] While pemoline failed to significantly reduce fatigue, a trend toward significance was seen at this higher dosage. Nineteen patients (46.3%) experienced excellent or good relief of fatigue with pemoline compared with eight patients (19.5%) on placebo ($P=0.06$). However, a significantly greater number of adverse effects was seen with pemoline compared with placebo, including irritability, insomnia, nausea, and anorexia. One quarter of the participants did not tolerate pemoline well, and 7% discontinued the drug due to intolerable adverse effects.[9]

Pemoline has been associated with several cases of life-threatening liver failure. Because of this, the drug's product labeling was updated in June 1999 to include a "black box" warning of this association.[12] For these reasons and the lack of strong efficacy data, pemoline use has been minimal, and is not generally recommended as a first-line therapy. For those in whom the drug is effective, it tends to work well, and some patients do prefer this medication. Its use should not be ruled out in patients who do not respond well to other medications.

Modafinil

Modafinil is a wake-promoting agent that is chemically and pharmacologically distinct from CNS stimulants. It is believed to work selectively in areas of the brain involved in the regulation of normal wakefulness (e.g., the hypothalamus).[13,14] This agent purportedly increases cortical activity by activating histaminergic pathways from the tuberomamillary nucleus,[14] although it is also likely that the agent works at least in part through dopaminergic pathways. The wake-promoting activity of modafinil has been studied in a number of clinical models, including narcolepsy,[15] obstructive sleep apnea,[16] chronic fatigue syndrome,[17] and as an adjunct therapy for depression.[18] Modafinil appears to be well tolerated; the most common adverse effects are headache, nausea, and nervousness. Unlike CNS stimulants such as methylphenidate and amphetamine, the potential for abuse appears to be lower,[19,20] which is reflected in its schedule IV labeling under the Controlled Substances Act (compared with schedule II labeling for methylphenidate and amphetamine). Safe long-term use has been documented in narcolepsy populations.[21]

The efficacy of modafinil for MS-related fatigue was evaluated in a 9-week, single-blind (to patients), forced titration trial of 72 patients with a mean FSS $\geqslant 4$.[10] The first 2 weeks of study served as a placebo run-in phase, followed by 2 weeks of modafinil 200 mg/day, 2 weeks of modafinil 400 mg/day, and a 3-week washout period. A number of scales commonly used to evaluate MS-related fatigue were employed, including the FSS, the Modified Fatigue Impact Scale (MFIS), and the VAS-F. The 200-mg dose of modafinil significantly improved fatigue compared with placebo at endpoint on all three of these scales (all $P<0.05$). Overall, 69% of patients experienced improvement with this dose on each of these scales. The drug was well tolerated, with the most common adverse events at the 200-mg dose being headache (17% versus 15% for placebo run-in), nausea (11% versus 6%), and anxiety (9% versus 1%). There was a high incidence of asthenia (14%) with the higher dose of 400 mg, which may be one of the reasons underlying the lack of significant effect with this dosage.

An open-label study of modafinil in 50 patients with relapsing-remitting or secondary progressive MS also showed a positive treatment effect.[22] The mean FSS score in this study was 30.3 at baseline (scores were calculated as the sum of the nine individual item scores). Treatment was started with a single daily modafinil dose of 100 mg, which was titrated in 100-mg increments based on efficacy and tolerability to a maximum daily dose of 400 mg.

Modafinil significantly improved fatigue, with the mean FSS score decreasing to 25.4 after 3 months ($P<0.0001$). On global response ratings, 44 patients reported either clear improvement or some improvement in their fatigue. Only three patients reported no change. Half of the patients remained on the 100-mg dose, with 42% increasing to 200 mg and 4% to 300 mg; no patient required 400 mg. Three patients discontinued modafinil use because of adverse events (nervousness and dizziness).

Antidepressants

Antidepressant medications have not been systematically studied for the management of MS-related fatigue. However, they are a vital intervention for the MS patient with depression and fatigue. In fact, it is appropriate to concentrate on a mood disorder if one is present before pursuing pharmacologic therapy for fatigue. Treatment of the fatigue first, without considering a strategy to alleviate mood disorders, can prove to be therapeutically ineffective.

The importance of controlling depression in the fatigue patient was illustrated in a clinical trial of 60 MS patients with moderate to severe depression who were randomized to antidepressant therapy, group psychotherapy, or behavioral therapy.[23] Patients were assessed at baseline using the Fatigue Assessment Instrument and Global Fatigue Severity subscale[24]; depression was assessed using the Beck Depression Inventory.[25] Fatigue severity was significantly reduced over the 16-week course of treatment ($P<0.02$), and this reduction was primarily attributed to the reduction achieved in depression scores.[23]

Additional evidence for antidepressant efficacy in the treatment of MS-related fatigue is available from two case reports in which improvements in energy and decreases in irritability were observed in MS patients treated with bupropion, started at 75–100 mg/day and increased to 200–300 mg/day in divided doses.[26] Sustained improvement in energy was seen over at least 6 months.

Given that fatigue is often associated with depression, and that depression is common in MS, there should be a willingness to aggressively treat signs and symptoms of depression in the MS patient. Because of their generally favorable safety profile, and because many of them are also indicated for treatment of anxiety, selective serotonin reuptake inhibitors or related antidepressant medications (such as the selective norepinephrine reuptake inhibitor bupropion) should be preferred over other classes of agents. Certain of these medications (e.g., fluoxetine, bupropion, and venlafaxine) are considered to have more "activating" properties than other antidepressant medications, and thus should be tried first.

Other Agents

Other agents that have been tried in the management of MS-related include the aminopyridines and transdermal histamine/caffeine. The aminopyridines (4-aminopyridine and 3,4-diaminopyridine) are potassium channel blockers that are used to prolong the duration of nerve action potential and improve the safety factor of nerve transmission.[27] They have been used successfully to overcome mobility problems such as transferring difficulties. A 1998 open-label study tested electrophysiologic parameters of motor performance in eight patients with a mean FSS score of 5.5. Significant subjective improvements in fatigue were reported with 3,4-diaminopyridine ($P<0.05$), but these did not correlate with significant improvements in electrophysiologic tests of motor conduction or other measures of motor function. The results were attributed to a potential nonspecific central stimulant effect of the medication.[27]

An earlier double-blind, crossover study had compared 3,4-diaminopyridine with 4-aminopyridine in 10 patients who were considered responders to 4-aminopyridine during a prior study by the researchers. Four of the patients were considered to have "clinically relevant changes" in fatigue with 4-aminopyridine as measured on a VAS, compared with only one patient on 3,4-diaminopyridine. Clinically relevant change was defined as a score on the VAS greater than the greatest change during treatment with 4-aminopyridine in the previous study.[28]

The aminopyridines are problematic in that they carry a high degree of seizure risk. Examples of major adverse events in studies of the aminopyridines were generalized seizures and hepatitis.[29] (In some investigations, patients are excluded if they have a history of seizures or significant electroencephalographic abnormalities.)[27] While these agents are currently not widely used, new formulations with improved safety profiles are under development, and are likely to become approved for clinical use to control neurologic symptoms such as spasticity. The availability of safer preparations of 4-aminopyridine will likely result in additional clinical research studies for individuals with MS.

A recent 12-week pilot study reported on the results of Prokarin™, a transdermal blend of histamine and caffeine.[30] A significant difference was seen between the 22 patients receiving Prokarin and the seven patients receiving placebo on MFIS scores (37.4 for active therapy versus 53.2 for placebo; $P<0.05$); this effect was seen at 4 weeks and continued throughout the 12-week duration of the study. No significant adverse events were reported with Prokarin use; however, there was a methodologic concern regarding how well matched the two groups were at baseline. Six of the seven placebo patients had a diagnosis of secondary or primary progressive MS, while only 13 of the 22 Prokarin patients had a progressive form of MS. Improvements in clinical trial design and better masking in larger trials are needed to validate these initial results.

Conclusions

If fatigue cannot be managed adequately through nonpharmacologic means, the overall body of evidence supports the use of amantadine and modafinil as first-line therapies in the management of MS-related fatigue. A recent consensus meeting of neurologists supported these conclusions, recommending amantadine as first-line therapy for mild fatigue (categorized as an FSS <4) and modafinil for more severe cases of fatigue (FSS ≥4) or for cases that have proved unresponsive to amantadine.[31] Because of the heterogeneity of MS fatigue and the substantial degree of impact on the patient, the physician should not hesitate to try other medications if the first does not appear to be effective. Monitoring medications used for other MS symptoms, such as spasticity and pain, should be performed to assess their potential impact on fatigue. For patients on interferon beta therapy, the degree of fatigue associated with the interferon injections should be assessed, and alternatives should be considered if fatigue proves severe, does not diminish over time, or is detrimental to the patient's functioning or well-being.

References

1. Multiple Sclerosis Council for Clinical Practice Guidelines. *Fatigue and Multiple Sclerosis: Evidence-Based Management Strategies for Fatigue in Multiple Sclerosis.* Washington, DC: Paralyzed Veterans Association; 1998.
2. Krupp LB, Christodoulou C, Madigan D, et al. The use of interferon beta-1a (IFN-beta-1a, Avonex) and modafinil to evaluate and treat cytokine-induced fatigue in multiple sclerosis. Presented at: the 127th Annual Meeting of the American Neurological Association; October 13-16, 2002; New York, NY.
3. Rio J, Nos C, Marzo ME, Tintore M, Montalban X. Low-dose steroids reduce flu-like symptoms at the initiation of IFNbeta-1b in relapsing-remitting MS. *Neurology.* 1998;50:1910-1912.
4. Copaxone® (glatiramer acetate injection) prescribing information. Kansas City, Mo: Teva Neuroscience; January 2002.
5. Murray TJ. Amantadine therapy for fatigue in multiple sclerosis. *Can J Neurol Sci.* 1985;12:251-254.
6. Cohen RA, Fisher M. Amantadine treatment of fatigue associated with multiple sclerosis. *Arch Neurol.* 1989;46:676-680.
7. Canadian MS Research Group. A randomized controlled trial of amantadine in fatigue associated with MS. *Can J Neurosci.* 1987;14:273-279.
8. Krupp LB, Coyle PK, Doscher C, et al. Fatigue therapy in multiple sclerosis: results of a double-blind, randomized, parallel trial of amantadine, pemoline, and

placebo. *Neurology*. 1995;45:1956-1961.

9. Weinshenker BG, Penman M, Bass B, Ebers GC, Rice GPA. A doubleblind, randomized, crossover trial of pemoline in fatigue associated with multiple sclerosis. *Neurology*. 1992;42:1468-1471.

10. Rammohan KW, Rosenberg JH, Lynn DJ, Blumenfeld AM, Pollak CP, Nagaraja HN. Efficacy and safety of modafinil (Provigil®) for the treatment of fatigue in multiple sclerosis: a two-centre phase 2 study. *J Neurol Neurosurg Psychiatry*. 2002;72:179-183.

11. Symmetrel® (amantadine) package insert. Chadds Ford, Pa: Endo Pharmaceuticals; May 2000.

12. Cylert® (pemoline) package insert. Chicago, III: Abbott Laboratories; June 1999.

13. Lin JS, Hou Y, Jouvet M. Potential brain neuronal targets for amphetamine-, methylphenidate-, and modafinil-induced wakefulness, evidenced by c-fos immunocytochemistry in the cat. *Proc Natl Acad Sci USA*. 1996;93:14128-14133.

14. Scammell TE, Estabrooke IV, McCarthy MT, et al. Hypothalamic arousal regions are activated during modafinil-induced wakefulness. *J Neurosci*. 2000;20:8620-8628.

15. US Modafinil in Narcolepsy Multicenter Study Group. Randomized trial of modafinil as a treatment for the excessive daytime somnolence of narcolepsy. *Neurology*. 2000;54:1166-1175.

16. Arnulf I, Homeyer P, Garma L, et al. Modafinil in obstructive sleep apnea-hypopnea syndrome: a pilot study in 6 patients. *Respiration*. 1997;64:159-161.

17. Cochran JW. Effect of modafinil on fatigue associated with neurological illnesses. *Journal of Chronic Fatigue Syndrome*. 2001;8:65-70.

18. Menza MA, Kaufman KR, Castellanos A. Modafinil augmentation of antidepressant treatment in depression. *J Clin Psychiatry*. 2000;61:378-381.

19. Jasinski DR. An evaluation of the abuse potential of modafinil using methylphenidate as a reference. *J Psychopharmacol*. 2000;14:53-60.

20. Rush CR, Kelly TH, Hays LR, Baker RW, Wooten AF. Acute behavioral and physiological effects of modafinil in drug abusers. *Behav Pharmacol*. 2002;13:105-115.

21. O'Malley M. Long-term safety and efficacy of modafinil for daytime sleepiness. Presented at: The 2002 Annual Meeting of the American Psychiatric Association; May 18-23, 2002; Philadelphia, Pa.

22. Zifko UA, Rupp M, Schwarz S, Zipko HT, Maida EM. Modafinil in the treatment of fatigue in multiple sclerosis: results of an open-label study. *J Neurol*. 2002;249:983-987.

23. Mohr DC, Hart SL, Goldberg A. Effects of treatment for depression on fatigue in multiple sclerosis. *Psychosom Med*. 2003;65:542-547.

24. Schwartz JE, Jandorf L, Krupp LB. The measurement of fatigue: a new instrument. *J Psychosom Res*. 1993;37:753-762.

25. Beck AT, Ward CH, Medelson M, Mock J, Erbaugh S. An inventory for measuring depression. *Arch Gen Psychiatry*. 1961;4:561-571.

26. Duffy JD, Campbell J. Bupropion for the treatment of fatigue associated with multiple sclerosis. *Psychosomatics*. 1994;35:170-171.

27. Sheean GL, Murray NM, Rothwell JC, et al. An open-labeled clinical and electrophysiological study of 3,4-diaminopyridine in the treatment of fatigue in multiple sclerosis. *Brain*. 1998;121:967-975.

28. Polman CH, Bertelsmann FW, de Waal R, et al. 4-aminopyridine is superior to 3,4-diaminopyridine in the treatment of patients with multiple sclerosis. *Arch Neurol*. 1994;51:1136-1139.

29. Polman CH, Bertelsmann FW, van Loenen AC, Koetsier JC. 4-aminopiridine in the treatment of patients with multiple sclerosis: long-term efficacy and safety. *Arch Neurol*. 1994;51:292-296.

30. Gillson G, Richards TL, Smith RB, Wright JV. A double-blind pilot study of the effect of Prokarin™ on fatigue in multiple sclerosis. *Mult Scler.* 2002;8:30-35.

31. Schapiro RT, for the The Working Group for Pharmacologic Therapy in Multiple Sclerosis-Related Fatigue. MS-related fatigue: toward a consensus for pharmacologic therapy. *Int J MS Care.* 2002;4(suppl):1-16.

Minimizing Fatigue by Conserving Energy

The following recommendations can be discussed with the patient as effective techniques to conserve energy during daily activities:

Overall Recommendations

- Balance activity with rest and learn to allow time to rest when planning a day's activity: *Rest means doing nothing at all*. There is a fine line between pushing to fatigue and stopping before it sets in. Rest improves endurance and leaves strength for enjoyable activities.
- Plan ahead: Make a daily or weekly schedule of activities to be done and spread heavy and light tasks throughout the day.
- Pace activity: Rest before you become exhausted. Taking time out for 5- or 10-minute rest periods during an activity may be difficult at first, but it may significantly increase overall functional endurance.
- Learn "activity tolerance": See if a given activity can be broken down into a series of smaller tasks or if others can assist in its performance.
- Set priorities: Focus on items that are priorities or that must be done, and learn to let go of guilt that may be associated with not finishing tasks as a result of fatigue.

Kitchen and Cooking Arrangements

- Store items that are used most often on shelves or in areas where they are within easy reach, to minimize the need to stretch and bend.
- Keep pots and pans near the stove, and dishes and glasses near the sink or eating area.
- Keep heavy appliances such as toasters and blenders in a permanent place on countertops.

- Have various working levels in the kitchen area to accommodate different tasks, and evaluate working heights to maintain good posture and prevent fatigue. Sit whenever possible while preparing meals or washing dishes, and use a large stool with casters that roll to eliminate at least some walking. When standing for a prolonged period, ease tension in your back by keeping one foot on a stepstool or an opened lower drawer.
- Use wheeled utility carts or trays to transport numerous and/or heavy items.
- Hang utensils on pegboards to provide easier accessibility.
- Have vertical partitions placed inside storage spaces to permit upright stacking of pots and pans, lids, and baking equipment.
- If storage cabinets are deep and hard to reach, use lazy Susans or sliding drawers to bring supplies and utensils within easy reach.
- Use cookware designed for oven-to-table use to eliminate the need for extra serving pieces. Use paper towels, plastic wrap, and aluminum foil to minimize cleanup.

Meal Preparation

- Have good lighting and ventilation in the cooking area.
- Gather items needed to prepare a meal, and then sit while doing the actual food preparation.
- Select foods that require minimal preparation—dehydrated, frozen, canned, or packaged mixes.
- Use a cutting board with nails to hold items that are being cut.
- Prepare double recipes, and freeze half for later use.
- Use electrical appliances rather than manual ones whenever possible, including food processors, mixers, blenders, and can openers.
- Use a microwave oven or crock pot to cut down on cooking and cleanup time.
- Bake rather than fry whenever possible.
- Bake cookies as sheets of squares instead of using shaped cutters.
- Slide heavy items along the countertop rather than lifting them.
- Use a damp dishcloth or a sticky substance such as Dycem™ to keep a pot or bowl in place while stirring.
- Line baking pans with foil to minimize cleanup, and soak pots and pans to eliminate scrubbing.

Cleaning

- Spread tasks out over a period of time; do one main job each day rather than an entire week's cleaning at one time.

- Alternate heavy cleaning tasks with light ones, and either get help or break major heavy duty cleaning tasks into several steps.
- Use a pail or basket to transport cleaning supplies from room to room to save on the number of trips back and forth.
- Use adaptive equipment, such as extended handles for dusters or brushes, to avoid bending.

Laundry

- Wash one or two loads as they accumulate rather than doing multiple loads less often.
- Collect clothes in one place, and transfer them to the laundry area in a wheeled cart if possible.
- If the laundry area is in a basement, plan to remain there until the laundry is done, and have a place to relax while you are waiting.
- If a clothesline is used, have it hung at shoulder height, and place the laundry basket on a chair while hanging laundry.
- Hang clothes promptly after they are dry to minimize ironing.
- Sit down while ironing.
- Buy clothes that require minimal maintenance.

Shopping for Groceries

- Plan menus before going to the store, and take a shopping list with you.
- Use the same grocery store on a regular basis, and learn where various items are located for easier shopping. Using a photocopied master grocery list that is organized to match the store layout is a simple way to minimize time and energy.
- Use home delivery whenever possible.

Bedroom Maintenance

- Put beds on rollers if they must be moved or keep them away from walls.
- Make one side of a bed completely, then finish the other side, to minimize the amount of walking involved.
- Organize closets for easy access by making top shelves and clothing rods low enough to reach without straining.
- Use lightweight storage boxes, hanging zippered clothes bags, and plastic boxes for items that are needed daily.

Yardwork

- Alternate tasks and incorporate short rest periods to avoid fatigue.

- Keep your garden small and easy to manage.
- Use adaptive equipment, such as handles with extensions, to minimize bending.

Infant and Child Care

- Always use your leg and arm muscles rather than your back muscles when lifting an infant or child.
- Wash, change, and dress an infant at counter height.
- Kneel while washing a child in a bathtub.
- Use disposable diapers.
- Adapt the fasteners on a child's clothing for easier dressing.
- Have a child stand on a footstool while helping him or her dress or wash.

Sitting and Desk Work

- Arrange your desk and chair heights to facilitate maintaining proper posture, to reduce slumping of the shoulders and neck flexion.
- Use a chair that has good back support.
- Arrange your office so that your file cabinets, computer terminal, and other equipment are easily accessible.
- Use small lazy Susans on the desktop for pens, paper clips, tape, stapler, etc.
- Use a phone device that allows the receiver to rest on your shoulder and frees your hands during extended conversations.

Dressing

- Lay out clothing for the next day before retiring.
- Sit while dressing whenever possible.
- When dressing, dress the weaker side first; when undressing, undress the strong side first.
- Use a long-handled shoe horn.

Bathing

- Organize shampoos, soaps, and toiletries, and keep them together by the bathtub or shower.
- Use grab bars to assist in safely getting in and out of the bathtub.
- Use a tub bench or stool while showering or bathing.
- Always avoid hot water while bathing because it increases fatigue.

Reprinted with permission from Schapiro RT. *Symptom Management in Multiple Sclerosis.* 4th ed. New York, NY: Demos Medical Publishing; 2003.

INDEX

Note: Boldface numbers indicate illustrations.